INTEGRATION OF HEALTH IN THE ELEMENTARY SCHOOL CURRICULUM

INTEGRATION OF HEALTH IN THE ELEMENTARY SCHOOL CURRICULUM

JAMES H. HUMPHREY

Nova Science Publishers, Inc.
Commack, New York

Editorial Production: Susan Boriotti
Office Manager: Annette Hellinger
Graphics: Frank Grucci and John T'Lustachowski
Information Editor: Tatiana Shohov
Book Production: Donna Dennis, Patrick Davin, Christine Mathosian, Tammy Sauter
and Diane Sharp
Circulation: Maryanne Schmidt
Marketing/Sales: Cathy DeGregory

Library of Congress Cataloging-in-Publication Data

Humphrey, James Harry, 1911-
     Integration of health in the elementary school school curriculum / by
     James H. Humphrey.
           p.   cm.
     Includes bibliographical references and index.
     ISBN 1-56072-514-1 .
     1. Health education (Elementary)--United States.
     2.Interdisciplinary approach in educaton--United States.
I. Title.
LB1588.U6H87   1997   97-41245
372.3'7--dc21   CIP

The authors and publisher haven taken care in preparation of this book, but make no
expressed or implied warranty of any kind and assume no responsibility for any errors or
omissions. No liability is assumed for incidental or consequential damages in connection
with or arising out of information contained in this book.

This publication is designed to provide accurate and authoritative information with regard
to the subject matter covered herein. It is sold with the clear understanding that the
publisher is not engaged in rendering legal or any other professional services. If legal or
any other expert assistance is required, the services of a competent person should be
sought. FROM A DECLARATION OF PARTICIPANTS JOINTLY ADOPTED BY A COMMITTEE
OF THE AMERICAN BAR ASSOCIATION AND A COMMITTEE OF PUBLISHERS.
Printed in the United States of America

CONTENTS

**CHAPTER 3   ARRANGEMENT OF HEALTH EDUCATION
                 CURRICULUM CONTENT   47**

**CHAPTER 4   TEACHING AND LEARNING APPLIED TO
                 HEALTH EDUCATION   65**

ABOUT THE AUTHOR

James H. Humphrey, Professor Emeritus at the University of Maryland has authored or coauthored more than 20 books about health and health education. He is a former Research Editor of *The Journal of School Health* and the first Chairman-Elect of the Research Council of the American School Association. He is the founder and editor of the research annual *Advances in Health Education: Current Research*. Dr. Humphrey has taught about health at all education levels from the elementary school through the University graduate level.

INTRODUCTION

It is the purpose of this text to include all of the elements needed to prepare elementary school teachers for the teaching of health. Thus, the book depicts the nature and structure of the school health program, proposes a health education curriculum suitable for the elementary school, presents principles of teaching methodology and emphasizes in detail specific ways in which health might be taught in other curriculum areas; that is, *integration*.

The titles of most of the chapters in this volume are self-explanatory. However, the matter of integration would seem to require special comment here. Integration has always been recommended as a very feasible way to include health teaching in the elementary school curriculum. For example, several decades ago the World Confederation of Organizations of the Teaching Profession reported that: "Educational authorities in the United States generally agree that health education at the elementary level should be integrated with all the other educational experiences and activities."

However, in spite of the many recommendations for using this approach in health teaching at the elementary school level, there is almost no literature which discusses integration techniques thoroughly. In this book, rather extensive treatment has been given to ways of integrating health and language arts, mathematics, science, social studies, physical education, and creative expression. It is hoped that the present material will shed additional light on how integration of health in the elementary school curriculum might be successfully accomplished: and it is hoped that it will encourage further experimentation with this procedure.

In order to provide for a better understanding of how health might be integrated with other areas of study, it appears necessary to discuss briefly the general nature of integration in education.

The term *integration* has taken on different meanings through the years, and as a consequence it may mean many different things to many different people. In simplest terms integration means the process of making whole. To integrate is to bring together the parts of the whole in order to derive some sort of functional unity.

An analysis of the literature suggests that educators appear to use the concept of integration in terms of the *psychological, sociological* and *educational* areas. The psychological aspect of integration concerns the total personality of the individual. This concept accepts the individual as a *total* being consisting of the highly interrelated and interdependent physical, social, emotional, and intellectual facets of personality.

Social integration is concerned with three different aspects. These include (1) the relationship between personalities, such as child with child and child with teacher; (2) the need for a desirable relationship between the individual and various agencies of society; and (3) consideration of the relationship between these various agencies of society.

The third concept, education integration, is the one that we are primarily concerned with here. This procedure involves teaching methods and techniques which relate and unify various subject-matter areas and skills through specific areas for the purpose of providing problem-solving as a way of learning. Educational integration tends to recognize that all areas of the curriculum in the elementary school in one way or another complement one another in the solution of problems for the learner.

Although modern educators have provided possibilities for the implementation of educational integration this concept is by no means news. For example, in the first century Marcus Fabius Quintilianus the renowned Roman rhetorician proclaimed, "Are we first to deliver ourselves up to the sole services of the teacher of literature, and then similarly to the teacher of geometry, neglecting under the latter what was taught us by the former?"

The extent to which the integration of health learning experiences with other curriculum areas is practiced in elementary schools is not entirely clear. Moreover, not too much is known about how successful this procedure has been in practical situations. My own research suggests that very few teachers are integrating health education activities into the elementary school program. The reason given for this is that there is a lack of information on how to carry out the process of integration. The degree of success that teachers have reported to me offers some evidence that health education activities afford an excellent medium for cooperative effort in utilizing the elementary school curriculum in a more functional way. Other results of my research seem to indicate that the integration of health education activities in the different parts of the curriculum may serve as a means of contributing simultaneously to the broader purposes of education. It has also revealed a need to explore further possibilities of integrating more health activities with other areas of the curriculum.

Finally, I should mention that I have been guided by the successful experiences of many outstanding elementary school classroom teachers, administrators, and supervisors with whom it has been my pleasure to associate through the years. In fact, these individuals provided much of the stimulus which resulted in the decision to prepare this volume. To them I wish to express my most sincere gratitude for the contributions, both direct and indirect, that they have made to the book.

CHAPTER 1

AN OVERVIEW OF SCHOOL HEALTH

An intelligent discussion of the sound treatment of any subject should perhaps begin with some sort of understanding of the terminology connected with that particular subject. This implies a consistent use of carefully defined terms as well as an insight into the relationship between certain terms. The many attempts to develop new definitions of old term and the introduction of new terms in certain fields have resulted, in some instances, in widespread confusion in the meaning and relationship of various commonly-used terms in these various fields. This widespread confusion in terminology exists in the area of *health*. I say this because I have had many inquiries over the years from parents and teachers with reference to the meaning of health and related terms. Such questions as "What is really meant by health?" seem to make it appropriate to devote a somewhat detailed discussion to this subject. To this end the terms *health* and *health education* will be described in the ensuing discussion.

THE MEANING OF HEALTH

Throughout the ages various scholars and philosophers have made pronouncements depicting the importance and meaning of health. Two examples of such citations are presented here: In 300 BC the Greek anatomist Herophilus, personal physician to Alexander the Great, postulated that when *health is absent, wisdom cannot reveal itself, art cannot become manifest, strength cannot fight, wealth becomes useless, and intelligence cannot be applied.* Centuries later Artur Schopenhauer (1788-1860), A German philosopher, proclaimed, *If you must waste money, time and health, do so in that order.*

In modern times, the precise meaning that one associates with the term *health* depends in a large measure on the particular frame of reference in which it is used. In recent years it was a relatively common practice to think of health in terms of the condition of the living organism that functioned normally. This idea about health is one that is still accepted by many people. In subscribing to this particular concept, these individuals tend to think of health predominantly as a state in which there is absence of pain or symptoms related to a poorly functioning organism. When thought of only in this manner, health is considered primarily in terms of a state in which there is absence of disease.

A modern concept considers health more and more in terms of *well-being*, which is perhaps the most important human value. In considering health from a point of view of well-being, the ideal state of health would be one in which all of the various parts of the human organism function at an optimum level at all times. This is perhaps what the notable American author and editor H.L. Mencken meant many years ago when he characterized the healthy man as one perfectly adjusted to his environment. Although it is very unlikely that the human organism will ever achieve the ideal state suggested here, such a level is ordinarily used as a standard for diagnosing or appraising the human health status.

The old meaning of health that considered it primarily only in terms of absence of disease tended to place it in a negative sense. The more modern concept places more positive emphasis on the term. This is to say that the meaning of health is interpreted as a level of well-being as well. It seems logical to assume that modern society's goal should be in the direction of achieving the highest level of well-being for all of its citizens, children as well as adults.

THE MEANING OF HEALTH EDUCATION

One meaning of the term *health education* that is becoming rather widespread describes it as *any purposeful effort that helps people to change their way of living to add years to life and life to years*. Thought of in these terms, health education might well be considered as an area where the specific purpose is teaching children how to live in a healthful and efficient way. In fact, health education could be one of the most important segments of American education because of its concern with teaching how to live well and how to get the most out of life. However, the question arises as to just how our citizenry is going to learn to live in a healthful manner. In the final analysis it will be up to education to prepare children to use the vast amount of health knowledge that has accumulated over the years. Therefore, the job of health education should be to provide desirable health learning experiences for children that will make it possible for them to make the most valid health decisions throughout their lives.

DIMENSIONS OF HEALTH EDUCATION

Health education is concerned with three important aspects. These are health *knowledge,* health *attitudes* and health *practices*. These areas may also be referred to as *domains* ; these are the *cognitive* domain (knowledge), the *affective* domain (attitudes), and the *action* domain (practices). Each of these dimensions will be dealt with separately in the ensuing discussion, but it appears important at the outset to consider them together for the purpose of a better understanding of how they are related.

In order for children to benefit most from the health learning experiences that are provided for them, it is most important that these experiences develop into desirable health practices. Thus, the ultimate goal should be in the direction of a kind of behavior that will be likely to insure optimum present and future health for the child. However, before the most desirable and worthwhile health practices can be achieved, there is a need for a certain amount of desirable health knowledge along with a proper attitude in making appropriate application of the knowledge to health practice.

Although it is obvious that to *know* is not necessarily to *do*; nevertheless, that which is done wisely will depend in a large measure upon the kind and amount of knowledge a child has acquired and the way in which health concepts are developed. In the accumulation of health knowledge the child will need to understand why it is beneficial for him or her to follow a certain practice. When the child does know why, it is perhaps more likely that there will develop a desirable attitude toward certain health practices. If a child has a sufficient amount of desirable health knowledge developed through valid health concepts, and also has a proper attitude, then he or she will be more apt to apply the knowledge to health behavior. Moreover, the child should be in a better position to exercise good judgment and make wise decisions in matters pertaining to health if the right kind and amount of health knowledge has been obtained.

HEALTH KNOWLEDGE (COGNITIVE DOMAIN)

Knowledge about health is acquired in a variety of different ways. Some of it is the product of tradition and, as such, oftentimes is nothing more than folklore. Certain popular notions about health related matters that have long since been dispelled are still held by many people who have not, for some reason or other, benefited from modern health knowledge. For example, for many years people subscribed to the notion that food left in a tin can after it was opened would become spoiled by contact with the tin. In reality, the food spoiled after opening the can as a result of bacterial growth rather than because of contact with the tin.

There are also many false notions about the health of children. A couple of examples of these untruths are reported here. The common belief about growing pains is incorrect. Although there may be muscle cramps, there is no such thing as pain caused by bone growth. Another widely accepted belief is that *all* boys and girls need a vitamin supplement to their regular diet. According to best authority, with the average American diet a healthy boy or girl does not need vitamin pills. The above examples and countless others that might be placed in the category of old wives' tales can be passed on from one generation to another if people fail to ask for scientific evidence to support such beliefs.

Other kinds of health knowledge of sorts are derived in our modern society from the constant bombardment of the eyes and ears of people through mass communication media such as television and radio. It is a known fact that a large percentage of television viewers are children. Although some of this information may be valid from a health point of view, people should, nevertheless, be alert to the possibility that the primary purpose of many kinds of advertising is to sell a product that proclaims results that are not likely to be attainable.

Another source of health knowledge is the home. In fact, most of our health learnings get their start in the home. Parents are our first teachers and, for better or for worse, what we learn from them mostly without our being aware of it tends to remain with us. A good home should contribute much to the health knowledge of its children simply by providing good meals, and a friendly, well-regulated, but pleasant and recreationally-challenging environment in which to grow up. Children from such homes ordinarily do not have to *un*learn a lot of faulty ideas and unwholesome attitudes when they are in the next potential source of health knowledge-the schools. It should be borne in mind that many children who grow up in homes in the inner city and some remote parts of the country do not benefit from good home health experiences and, thus, their *first* source of health knowledge is the school.

In recent years there has been a growing recognition of the fact that if people are going to be healthy they must obtain valid knowledge in health matters. The providing of such knowledge appears to be a very important function of the nation's schools. Because the schools are organized in such a way as to provide a climate for desirable learning, boys and girls can be placed in problem-solving situations and be taught *why* certain things are important to their health. For example, if one is required to eat foods that are good for him or her but is never taught *why*, it is important that the child be taught so that when away from the control of parents he or she will not tend to choose foods entirely on the basis of what tastes best, but will take into account the needs of the body. Moreover, if a child has never been taught what constitutes a good diet, it is not likely that he or she will know how to select one even if at last becoming aware of the importance of a good diet for vigorous health, weight control and body efficiency. Thus, it should be seen that knowledge in health matters requires good teaching in a desirable educational setting.

The scope of knowledge that one might obtain about matters related to health is almost endless, and obviously it would be difficult to learn all there is to know about it. However, there are certain basic concepts about health that should be developed by boys and girls at all age levels. Generally speaking, the individual should acquire knowledge pertaining to the direct basic needs of the human organism, and, in addition, knowledge regarding the human organism as it functions in its environment. (This will be discussed in detail in the following chapter.)

As indicated at the outset of this discussion, health knowledge may be derived from many sources. Some are valid and some are not. It remains for education to help the individual sort out the truths from the untruths and, hence, to act accordingly in the best interest in his or her own health and that of society as a whole.

The age old adage "knowledge is power" is certainly applicable to knowledge about health. When such knowledge is provided under suitable learning conditions, the individual should be empowered to live a fuller and happier life.

HEALTH ATTITUDES (AFFECTIVE DOMAIN)

Any discussion of attitudes requires an identification of the meaning of the term. Although it is recognized that different people will attach different meanings to the term *attitude*, for purposes here attitude will be thought of as being associated with *feelings*. We hear such expressions as How do you *feel* about it? In a sense, this implies What is your *attitude* toward it? Therefore, theoretically at least, attitude could be considered a factor in the determination of action because of this feeling about something. For example, knowledge alone that exercise is beneficial rarely leads to regular exercising, but a strong feeling or attitude might be a determining factor that leads one to exercise regularly.

It should be mentioned at this point that, contrary to abundant empirical thought, there is little or no objective evidence to support unequivocally the contention that attitude has a positive direct influence on behavior. One of the difficulties in studying this phenomenon scientifically lies in the questionable validity of instruments used to measure attitudes. Moreover, there is no consistent agreement with regard to the meaning of attitudes. Thus, the position taken here is one of theoretical postulation based upon logical assumption.

As far as health attitudes are concerned, they could well be considered a gap that can possibly exist between health knowledge and health practice, and this gap needs to be bridged if effective health behavior is to result from acquiring valid health knowledge.

In the school situation the development of proper attitudes is ordinarily considered to be primarily a function of the teacher. However true this may be the point of view taken here is that is also essential that the child be given an opportunity to accept a degree of the responsibility for attitude development. This should not be interpreted to mean that the teacher is free of such responsibility, but, on the other hand, the child should be made aware of the fact that he or she has the ability to associate feelings with thoughts and ideas that are acquired from the teacher. However, this association of feelings with ideas will be present even if the teacher gives it little or no attention.

In illustrating some of the above comments, let us say that a sixth grade boy has acquired some knowledge regarding the degree to which cigarette smoking can be harmful to health. Perhaps he will have some sort of underlying feeling toward such knowledge. He may choose to disregard it because some of his friends have also assumed such an attitude toward it, or he may feel that the evidence is convincing enough for him to believe that cigarette smoking is something he can get along without. In either case he has developed an attitude toward the practice of cigarette smoking and may react in accordance with this feeling. It should also be mentioned that he may not necessarily react in accordance with his own feelings because he may consider it fashionable or grown-up to smoke cigarettes so as not to lose status with friends who do. Whatever way he chooses to react will be tempered at least to an extent by the consequences that he associates with the knowledge he has acquired about cigarette smoking. Incidentally, we know of one particular sixth grader, who upon the acquisition of some knowledge about smoking and lung cancer, commented that by the time he was grown there would probably be a cure for lung cancer so smoking cigarettes would not make any difference. To say the least, such unaltering faith and desultory attitudes present a challenge to most elementary school teachers.

Obviously, one would hope that the accumulation of health knowledge would be accompanied by a positive attitude, and that this attitude would result in desirable action. It is possible that only in terms of such a positive attitude are desirable health practices and, hence, a better way of living likely to result. It should go without saying that the key figure in this process is the teacher.

HEALTH PRACTICE (ACTION DOMAIN)

It was suggested previously that to *know* is not necessarily to *do*. It is a well-known fact that all people do not capitalize on the knowledge they have acquired. Perhaps many children are apt to act only on impulse; actions of others are influenced to an extent by their friends. However, in a matter as important as one's health, it appears that a reasonable course to follow would be one in which the individual weighs the facts and scientific evidence before acting, but this is much easier for adults than for children.

Perhaps we might look at health practices that are desirable and those that are undesirable, or, in other words, those health practices that will result in pleasantness or unpleasantness. If we weigh knowledge in these terms, then perhaps we can appreciate better the possible consequences of certain health practices.

To change behavior is not always an easy matter. However, teachers are hopeful that children will modify their own health behavior after acquiring desirable health knowledge and forming favorable health attitudes. Although education may be compulsory to a certain age level, at the same time it is not necessarily *compulsion*. This is to say, in a sense, that while the school may provide a desirable setting for learning about health, in the final analysis the individual will make the decisions regarding his or her own health practices. In younger children this notion is impractical if we expect the best learning to take place; and forcing health practices upon children as they grow older not only appears impractical, but, in many cases, unwarranted as well.

As far as one's personal health is concerned, it perhaps becomes a matter of how much risk one is willing to take, and health practices are likely to be based upon this factor. By way of illustration let us refer again to cigarette smoking and health. There has been a great deal of information accepted as evidence from a medical point of view that indicates that smoking can contribute to certain types of serious diseases. Yet, many individuals are willing to assume a dangerous risk in defiance of such evidence.

After a person has learned about some aspect of health he or she is left with an element of choice. It is hoped that one would choose a course of health action that would involve a minimum of risk. Health education does not attempt to *control* the behavior of the individual, but to provide him or her with the knowledge needed to make the best possible decisions as far as health behavior is concerned.

SCOPE OF THE SCHOOL HEALTH PROGRAM

Although the major focus of this book is on health teaching in the elementary school, it nevertheless seems appropriate that the prospective teacher be given some insight into the various aspects of the total school health program. The main purpose of this, of course, is to give the reader some understanding of how health teaching relates to the other aspects of the school health program as well as to indicate what the teacher's responsibilities are in the larger area of school health.

It might be well to bring to the attention of the reader at this point the fact that the field of school health is characterized by the somewhat unusual distinction of having a proposed list of standardized terms. This is mentioned here because the scope of the various areas of school health alluded to throughout this text might be better understood if these areas are specifically defined.

Attempts at standardization of terminology in school health began over half a century ago through the efforts of the Health Education Section of the American Physical Education Association. Through the years many of the health education areas took on new meanings which made it necessary to redefine terms and clarify certain features in school health. The Committee on Terminology in School Health of the American Alliance for Health, Physical Education, Recreation and Dance has carried out this function over the years.

The terminology and definitions of the various areas of school health used throughout this volume will be based as far as possible upon recommendations of this committee. However, it should be borne in mind that attempts to standardize terminology in such a rapidly changing and expanding area as school health precludes a static list of standardized terms. Consequently, terminology and descriptions or definitions of the various areas of school health will deviate from the committee's recommendations as seems necessary in terms of present theories and practices.

It is a generally accepted idea that the total *school health program* involves those procedures that contribute to the understanding, maintenance and improvement of the health of children and school personnel. In carrying out these functions the total school health program is composed of three areas: *school health service, school health environment* and *school health education*. These three areas are interrelated and, to a large extent, interdependent; they are, however, obviously separate enough to warrant individual discussions.

SCHOOL HEALTH SERVICE

School health service attempts to conserve, protect, and improve the health of the school population. This objective is achieved in part through such procedures as (1) appraising the health status of children and school personnel; (2) counseling with children, parents and others involved in the appraisal findings; (3) helping to plan for the health care and education of exceptional children; (4) helping to prevent and control disease; and (5) providing for emergency care for sick and injured children.

The maximum function of school health service should provide all necessary health supervision to arrive at optimal health for all children. Naturally, such service depends upon the availability of specialized personnel such as physicians, dentists, nurses, psychologists and others who can make worthwhile contributions to the health of children. The type of extent of service that is actually provided in a given school system also depends upon such factors as available funds, size of school enrollment and availability of properly trained personnel. Because of these factors, the range of school health services varies markedly from one school system to another.

The extreme importance of the health service aspect of the school health program is obvious when one considers the range of anomalous health conditions of the school population. For instance, some estimates indicate that, on the average, out of every one hundred children of school age, one has heart disease, 20 have visual disorders, 10 have some degree of growth problems, 85 have dental disease and 20 have emotional disturbances. Added to these estimates are the fact that many children are only partially immunized and countless others live under conditions of poor health practices that involve lack of sleep, fresh air and sunshine.

Adequate school health services can do much to help eliminate these conditions. This is particularly true at the elementary school level because the younger the child is at the time a deviation from normal health is discovered, the greater the opportunity for proper care and possible recovery.

ROLE OF THE CLASSROOM TEACHER IN SCHOOL HEALTH SERVICE

Depending upon certain factors previously mentioned, the function of the classroom teacher in the school health service will vary from one school system to another. However, there are certain types of responsibilities that classroom teachers will likely be expected to assume in most elementary schools. One of the major responsibilities is concerned with the health appraisal of children. Since teachers are in daily contact with children, coupled with their knowledge of growth and development, they are in an excellent position to note changes in appearance and behavior that are associated with a child's health status. When a teacher detects something that indicates a deviation from the normal health status, a referral can be made to the proper person in the health service (ordinarily the school nurse) who can follow up the referral.

The responsibility for continually observing children for evidences of departure from health and the making of suitable referrals does not carry with it the further responsibility of diagnosing specific illnesses. Diagnosis is a matter that rests with medical, psychological, speech and other specialists. However, the more detailed and accurate the teacher's noting of pertinent symptoms, the more valuable the information he or she can provide to those responsible for diagnosis.

Acute illnesses, such as the onset of measles and appendicitis usually attract attention quickly and offer relatively little difficulty in the way of diagnosis to qualified specialists. On the other hand, the less abrupt departures from health, such as growth failure due to certain diseases or malnutrition, and some behavior disorders in the emotional life of the child, tend to offer greater diagnostic difficulties.

Information that the teacher may provide may be of considerable value in identifying the nature of the child's problem. For example, the teacher may give details about a particular child's increased irritability, reduced vitality, or tendency to withdraw from activities which might not be apparent in an interview or medical examination but which might be important factors in general health appraisal.

The following outline of signs and symptoms is presented merely as a guide to common indications of trouble in regard to child health.

1. *Facial Appearance.* The facial appearance of the child frequently gives an indication of present status. One should be alert to such symptoms as: unusual redness or pallor of the face, inflammation of the eyeballs, and a running nose. Such signs individually or in combination, can be brought on by various diseases, but in any event they are common signs of trouble and should receive attention. Although these symptoms signal the onset of common respiratory illnesses, they are also symptoms of some of the more severe diseases of children.

2. *The Respiratory System.* Respiratory diseases are the principal cause of absenteeism among children and although they are not usually very severe, in some cases they are quite serious. Colds and other respiratory disturbances are thought to be most contagious in their early stages; that is, within the first two or three days. Since many more serious diseases may resemble a simple cold in their early stages, the child should be watched closely for evidence of mounting fever, muscular pain, nausea, and other symptoms. Although there are not at present very effective means of curing colds, children should be

taught the importance of wearing proper clothing, eating wisely and getting enough rest in order to keep the frequency and severity of colds to a minimum.

Teachers can easily check mouth breathers to determine whether they are unable to breathe through the nose freely. Inability to breathe easily through the nose is indicative of some form of nasal blockage which should receive medical consideration.

Special note should be made of those individuals who are subject to repeated colds and suitable referrals should be made. Frequent colds may be indicative of a dietary deficiency, some chronic infection, poor dressing habits, or other factors related to a lowered resistance. They may also be related to a disturbed state in the emotional life of the child.

3. *The Eyes.* Certain behavior patterns should give rise to suspicion that the eyes are not functioning properly. For example, a child may hold reading material within a few inches of the face, may squint and make faces as he or she strains to read what is on the chalkboard. One's eyes may be very sensitive to light and he or she may wipe or rub the eyes frequently or close one eye when trying to see. Upon being questioned, the child may complain of blurred vision, headache and dizziness when reading or doing close work, or of not being able to see the ball or other objects when playing games. In appearance, the eyes may be watery and inflamed and the lids swollen and encrusted.

Glasses to not always assure correction of visual defects. When children with glasses show signs of visual difficulty, it is well to bear in mind the possibilities that diagnosis may not have been correct and the glasses do not provide the necessary compensation, or that the new difficulties have developed since the previous diagnosis.

The teacher can play an important role in encouraging children to wear their glasses, since it sometimes happens that they refuse to wear them for fear of being teased or appearing "different". Skillful teaching can help to make glasses socially acceptable among children.

4. *The Ears.* Partial hearing loss can frequently be identified by certain typical behaviorisms of children. They may strain forward with an intent look when instructions are being given, turn one ear toward the speaker or cup a hand behind the ear. If a child cannot hear his or her own voice well, the

speech may become flat and poorly modulated. It sometimes happens that children who appear dull or disinterested in class activities are merely unable to hear clearly what is taking place.

5. *The Neck.* Lumps in the neck may be due to mumps which cause a swelling of the salivary glands or to swelling of the lymph nodes just below the ear and behind the jaw. Lumps of either kind should receive the attention of a physician. Swelling of the lymph nodes indicates the presence of infection, perhaps in the gland itself or in some other region of the head, the ear, or throat.

6. *The Throat.* Dental screening in schools oftentimes reveals that approximately 80 percent or more of the children are in need of treatment. Although a satisfactory evaluation of dental health requires trained personnel, there are certain gross symptoms that the teacher should recognize. Some of these are: in very bad cases it is possible to see the dark yellow spots of decay at the base and sides of the front teeth; sometimes the foul smell of infection may be perceptible on the child's breath; the gums may be inflamed and sore; and the very obvious symptoms of toothache.

7. *The Hair and Scalp.* Ringworm is a condition that may be recognized by the forming of nearly bald areas and crustiness of the scalp. It can spread rapidly from child to child.

Pediculi or lice usually appear in regions where living conditions are unhygienic, but they may spread rapidly to anyone who is nearby. The teacher should be able to recognize the pests and become suspicious when the small eggs or nits are discovered clinging to the hair. Frequent itching of the scalp should be investigated for disease or infestation.

8. *Posture.* Poor posture may take several forms such as the head carried too far forward, round shoulders, one shoulder held higher than the other, sway back or forward curvature of the spine, pronated ankles, and flat fleet. The poor posture of some children is due to actual deformation of the skeleton and treatment is necessarily a medical matter. Most cases of poor posture are functional and due to difficulties other than skeletal abnormality.

It should be recognized that although poor posture may be due to bad habits of sitting, standing, and moving, or to the influence of unfortunate fads and styles, it is frequently a symptom of some underlying difficulty. Therefore it is unwise to require children to begin taking exercises or other corrective measures. For example, it would plainly be unwise to initiate an exercise program for a round shouldered boy if his stance is due to weakness from disease or malnutrition. Similarly, it would be unwise to suggest corrective activities to a child whose head-forward stance represents an attempted compensation for poor vision which actually can only be corrected by glasses. It is known, too, that prolonged emotional upset can be a cause of poor posture, and that improvement must begin with relieving the disturbing situation.

Once underlying causes of poor posture have been removed, the task is to convince the child as to the advantages of good posture and to guide his or her self-analysis so that improvement can take place. Whatever its cause, poor posture may become a habit which is broken only with conscious effort. Therefore, it is plain that children must want good posture if improvement is to take place.

Among very young children, improved use of the feet may result from teaching them to walk and run with the toes pointing forward. Older children can appreciate the principles of body mechanics involved. Of course, severe cases should be referred to a physician for evaluation and possible treatment.

The teacher's guidance can also be of great importance in the matter of selecting proper footwear. Children should be taught to have their feet properly measured and fitted; and they should be taught the hazard to their feet of wearing shoes that are in poor repair. For example, as a heel becomes worn on the inside, additional body weight is thrown upon the inside of the foot and there is increased tendency towards protonation or forcing the ankle inward and downward.

9. *Speech Difficulties.* Speech defects should be mentioned because of their frequency, oftentimes in combination with hearing loss. The full implication of speech defects cannot be appreciated until they are considered in the light of (1) their obvious interference with the most essential of our communication media, (2) the impact that they tend to have upon the emotions of the individual who possesses them, both because of the defective communication and because of the typical parental and other social reactions to them, and (3) the role that emotional upset commonly plays in the formation of speech defects.

Speech difficulties should be approached with caution because inept handling may complicate and aggravate rather than improve them. One specialist on speech once pointed out that most speech problems have their start, not in the mouths of children but in the mouths of their parents. This statement suggests that emotional problems are intimately involved in the speech situation, and it is likely that therapy in specific cases involves more than practicing saying words or being reminded not to stutter. As a matter of fact, the teacher who has not had specialized training in the area of speech therapy should realize that this difficulty, like a physical or mental disorder, is best left to a specialist.

Another likely responsibility of the classroom teacher in school health service is that which is concerned with emergency illness or injury. Ideally all school personnel should have an understanding of how to care for a child in case of a sudden illness or injury. It is particularly important that the classroom teacher have the skills necessary to render first aid. One of the most important factors in this regard is a teacher's full understanding of the school's policy regarding emergency care. With such knowledge at hand, the teacher can administer first aid as set forth in the prescribed school policy.

SCHOOL HEALTH ENVIRONMENT

This aspect of the school health program involves procedures that provide for the most satisfactory living conditions within the school plant and surrounding areas. A healthful school environment is concerned with (1) organizing the school day on a basis commensurate with the health and safety of children, and (2) providing for physical aspects of the school plant-proper ventilation, heating, lighting and the other aspects that are essential for preservation of an optimum health status.

As in the case of school health service, there is likely to be a wide range of standards of a school health environment among school systems. The standard that a given school system provides will be governed largely by available funds and specialized personnel, particularly in the area of school maintenance.

Everyone in the school system should take some degree of responsibility for ensuring a satisfactory school health environment. The position of leadership in individual schools is, of course, that of the school principal. His or her awareness of the meaning of a healthful school environment and how to implement it depends, to a considerable extent, upon the success of this aspect of the school health program.

Although there is no question that the principal's leadership is of prime importance to the satisfactory conducting of this environmental aspect of the school health program, the importance of other personnel should not be underestimated. Thus, classroom teachers play a major role in seeing that they and their children participate in a satisfactory manner in the program. Moreover, the teacher is in an ideal position to keep the school administration sensitive to new problems and developments that require action that is beyond the teacher's scope or that of any individual class.

The children of the school, too, should be considered active participants in the maintenance of a healthful school environment, and, of course, the teacher can use this part of the school health program as a means of conveying basic principles of cleanliness and sanitation that are important to group living.

The role of certain other personnel in the maintenance of a healthful school environment is so obvious as to require only brief mention in rounding out the total picture. Doctors, nurses, custodial staffs, food service personnel and public health officials are all vitally concerned. Also on occasion, problems may arise that require the attention of parent-teacher organizations as well as certain professional groups in the community.

SCHOOL HEALTH EDUCATION

It is the purpose of this aspect of the school health program to provide desirable and worthwhile learning experiences that will favorably influence knowledge, attitudes and practices pertaining to individual and group health. The medium through which these experiences can best be provided is health teaching. It is this phase of the school health program with which this book is primarily concerned. Subsequence chapters will deal extensively with the most accepted procedures for teaching elementary school children about health with particular emphasis upon integration.

Without disputing the importance or even the indispensability of school health services and school health environment, it must be emphasized that health teaching which is designed to increase the individual's ability to live healthily and deal intelligently with his or her own health problems is basic to the whole concept of healthful living. Although some efforts are being made to procure more special teachers it is quite clear that the major responsibility for health teaching in the elementary school will rest with the classroom teacher. However, in many situations the teacher has numerous resources to draw upon the way of materials and various health and safety personnel connected with either the school or the local public health organization. The teacher is responsible for utilizing these in such a way that they fit into the sequence of learning experiences.

Recognition of the importance of health teaching during the early years of life has gradually result in a national tendency to place greater emphasis upon health in the curriculum at all grade levels. More and more schools are making a definite effort to cover a series of health topics that are considered vital to the present and future health of the child. Many states have laws requiring that certain health topics be presented. These required topics were at first quite limited, commonly amounting to the effects of alcohol, tobacco and narcotics upon the body. However, for many years there has been a definite trend to go far beyond teaching only those health topics required by the old laws.

QUALIFICATIONS OF TEACHERS

There are certain *general* abilities required for teaching in any of the subject areas, and teaching about health in the elementary school does not differ extensively from teaching in the other curriculum areas. On the other hand, it should be recognized that by the very nature of the content of some curriculum areas, *specific* abilities may be needed for teachers to be most successful in certain areas. This is no doubt true in the area of health teaching. While an understanding of children should certainly be a general requirement for all teachers, the need for it is perhaps even more pronounced in the area of health because health-teaching content is inherently involved in understanding the child and how he or she learns.

UNDERSTANDING THE CHILD

As the child progresses through various stages of growth and development, certain distinguishing characteristics can be identified that suggest implications for effective teaching and learning about health.

The range of age levels from five through seven years usually includes children from kindergarten through second grade. During this period the child begins his or her formal education. In our culture the child leaves the home for a part of the day to take his or her place in a classroom with children of approximately the same chronological age. Not only is the child taking an important step toward becoming increasingly more independent and self-reliant, but learning takes place as he or she moves from being a highly self-centered individual to becoming a more socialized member of the group.

This stage is ordinarily characterized by a certain lack of motor coordination because the small muscles of the hands and fingers are not as well developed as the large muscles of the arms and legs. Thus, as the child starts formal education there is a need to use large crayons or pencils as one means of expression. The urge to action is expressed through movement since the child lives in a movement world so to speak. Children at these age levels thrive on vigorous activity. They develop as they climb, run, jump, hop, skip or keep time to music. An important physical aspect at this level is that the eyeball is increasing in size and the eye muscles are developing. This factor is an important determinant in the child's readiness to see and read small print, and, thus, it involves a sequence from large print on charts to primer type in preprimers and primers.

Even though the child has a relatively short attention span, he or she is extremely curious about the environment. At this stage the teacher can capitalize upon the child's urge to learn by providing opportunities to gain information from firsthand experiences through the use of the senses. He or she sees, hears, smells, feels and even tastes in order to learn. For instance, the child learns about the different parts of plants that we eat (root, stem, leaf) through actually handling and examining fruits and vegetables.

The age range from eight to nine years is the period that usually marks the time spent in the third and fourth grades. The child now has a wider range of interests and a longer attention span. While strongly individualistic, he or she is working more from a position in a group. Organized games should afford opportunities for developing and practicing skills in good leadership and followship as well as body control, strength and endurance. Small muscles are developing, manipulative skills are increasing and muscular coordination is improving. The eyes have developed to a point where the child can, and does, read more widely. He or she is capable of getting information from books and is beginning to learn more through vicarious experience. However, experiments carry an impact for learning at this age by capitalizing upon the child's curiosity. This is the stage of development when skills of communication (listening, speaking, reading and writing) and the number system are needed to deal with situations both in and out of school.

During the ages of ten through twelve most children complete the fifth and sixth grades. This is a period of transition for most as they go from childhood into the preadolescent period of growth and development. They may show concern over bodily changes and are sometimes self-conscious about appearance. At this range of age levels children tend to differ widely in physical maturation and in emotional stability. Greater deviations in growth and development can be noted within the sex groups than between them. Rate of physical growth can be rapid, sometimes showing itself in poor posture and restlessness. Some of the more highly organized team games such as softball, modified soccer and the like help furnish the keen and wholesome competition desired by these children. It is essential that the teacher recognize that, at this level, prestige among peers is more important than adult approval. During this period the child is ready for a higher level of intellectual skills which involve reasoning, discerning fact from opinion, noting cause-and-effect relationships, drawing conclusions and using various references to locate and compare the validity of information. He or she is beginning to show more proficiency in expression through oral and written communication.

Thus, during the years between kindergarten and the completion of sixth grade, the child grows and develops (1) socially, from a self-centered individual to a participating member of a group; (2) emotionally, from a state manifesting anger outbursts to a higher degree of self-control; (3) physically, from childhood to the brink of adolescence; and (4) intellectually, from learning by firsthand experience to learning from more technical and specialized resources.

If the child is to be educated as a growing organism, aspects of growth and development need the utmost consideration of the teacher in planning and guiding the health-learning activities which will be most profitable for the child at a particular stage of development.

SUGGESTIONS FOR SUPPLEMENTARY READING

Aronson, S.S., New recommendations for child check-ups and Winter brings strep throats, *Child Care Information Exchange*, 106, November/December 1995, p. 72-3.

Bradley, B.J., The school nurse as health educator, *The Journal of School Health*, 67, January 1997, p. 3-8.

Caughy, M.O., Health and environmental effects on the academic readiness of school-age children, *Developmental Psychology*, 32, May 1996, p. 512-22.

Coleman, E., Health-related knowledge: where does it come from?, Journal of Biological Education, 29, Summer 1995, p. 139-46.

Francis, E.E., et al., Who dispenses pharmaceuticals to children at school? *The Journal of School Health*, 66, December 1996, p. 355-8.

Humphrey, J.H., *Supervision in Health Education*, Springfield, IL, Charles C. Thomas Publisher, 1994, p. 3-8.

Humphrey, J.H., *Elementary School Child Health*, Springfield, IL, Charles C. Thomas Publisher, 1993, p. 18-24, 58-60.

Shaw, S.R., et al, School-linked and school-based services: a renewed call for collaboration between school psychologists and medical professionals, *Psychology in the Schools*, 32, July 1995, p. 190-201.

Ubbes, V.A., Promoting healthful behaviors in children and youth, *Journal of Health Education*, 27, September/October 1996, p. 58-9.

Welle, H.M., et al, Philosophical trends in health education: implications for the 21st century, *The Journal of School Health*, 26, November/December 1995, p. 326-32.

CHAPTER 2

SELECTION OF HEALTH EDUCATION CURRICULUM CONTENT

This chapter is concerned with *bases for selecting what to teach in the area of health*. That is, the most desirable and worthwhile learning experiences that should be provided for elementary school children. In this regard, the following two concerns should be taken into account: *principles of health education curriculum development* and *criteria for the selection of health education curriculum content*.

SOME BASIC PRINCIPLES OF HEALTH EDUCATION CURRICULUM DEVELOPMENT

It seems essential that those persons responsible for curriculum development in health education be guided by certain rules of action in order to avoid unnecessary pitfalls. The list of principles suggested here is perhaps by no means all-inclusive. Neither is each principle a separate entity. On the other hand, it may be noted that they overlap to some extent and, as a consequence, serve the purpose of integration and interrelation of the basic considerations essential to the success of the school health education program.

1. *The health education curriculum should comprise all of the experiences that children have in this area that are under the auspices of the school.* This principles implies that each component part of the program is interrelated with and dependent upon the other parts. The point of view is taken that school

health service, and school health environment provide, at least, indirect health learning experiences for children.

2. *Health education curriculum development should be based on a philosophy of equal opportunity for all children.* Health education is the rightful heritage of all of the children in all of the schools. If principles of democracy are to be practiced in the public schools of America, health education programs must be devised so that all children will have an equal opportunity to engage in wholesome health education experiences.

3. *Health education curriculum development should exhaust all of the available resources of the school and community.* It is incumbent upon the person in charge of school health education to survey each available resource and evaluate its possible use in school health education. In other words, this person along with teachers and others should investigate all possibilities that lend themselves to a more adequate and complete school health education program.

4. *Curriculum development should be a cooperative enterprise.* The time is past when health education curriculum development should be placed in the hands of a single individual. The cooperation of supervisors, teachers and others in providing worthwhile health education learning experiences for children is perhaps one of the best known means of improving the teacher-child learning situation in health education. Consequently, supervisors, teachers and others should pool their knowledge and experience in an attempt to develop a program that will make significant contributions to the optimum growth and development of children.

5. *Health education curriculum development recognizes individual differences in children.* In order to develop each individual to his or her ultimate capacity, health education curriculum development must take into consideration the fact that children differ with respect to physical, social, emotional and intellectual characteristics. Such factors as classification of children must be regarded as highly significant if the school plans to assume the responsibility for the optimum health learning of each individual child.

6. *Health education curriculum planning should be flexible.* The curriculum should be characterized by a degree of flexibility. Varying backgrounds of previous child experiences, particularly in the home, in health

education activities manifests a need for a curriculum that can be adapted to meet the specific needs of the children of a particular school.

7. *Health education curriculum should be continuous.* Since education is considered as a continuous process, it naturally follows that health education curriculum development should be continuous in order to meet the needs of a changing society.

CRITERIA FOR THE SELECTION OF HEALTH EDUCATION CURRICULUM CONTENT

Although various valid criteria might be considered as bases for selecting health curriculum content it appears sufficient here to deal only with the two broad general criteria of health *needs* and health *interests* of children.

RELATIONSHIP OF HEALTH NEEDS AND HEALTH INTERESTS

The terms *needs* and *interests* of children have been used together so often that there is a strong likelihood that their meanings have become confused. For this reason it appears important that the ensuing discussion be prefaced by a few comments about the relationship of needs and interests.

In thinking of terms of their relationship one must also consider how they differ. While health needs and interests of children may be closely related and highly interdependent, there are nevertheless certain important differences that should be taken into account when these criteria are used as bases for the selection of health curriculum content.

Needs of children, particularly those of an individual nature, are likely to be innate. On the other hand, interests for the most part may be acquired as products of the environment. Herein lies a different of paramount importance in the selection of health curriculum content for children of elementary school age. For example, it is possible that a child may demonstrate an interest in a certain unsafe practice that is obviously not compatible with his or her needs at a certain age level. The two-year old may be interested in running into the street, but this practice might result in injury. Acquisition of a particular interest because of environmental conditions is further illustrated in the case of children coming from families who might be superstitious about certain kinds of foods, or of certain foods eaten in combination. In such cases the acquisition of such an interest from other family members might build up a lifetime resistance to a certain kind of food that might be very nutritious and beneficial to the child's physical needs.

Perhaps one of the most important aspects involved in the relationship between health needs and health interests is that of obtaining a proper ratio between the two. Arriving at a happy medium between needs and interests is at best a very difficult problem. We should think first in terms of meeting the child's health needs, but we need interest in order for the most desirable learning to take place. Consequently, when health needs and interests are combined in proper ratio, a near-ideal situation exists for desirable and worthwhile learning about health.

In determining the degree of health needs and interests as criteria for health curriculum content we might well be guided by the age levels of children. In this regard a general principle is that the lower the age level of children the more we can depend upon health needs as a valid criterion. This is based on the assumption that the younger the child the less experience he or she has had, and consequently there is less opportunity to develop certain interests. In other words, a lack of interest at an early age level might possibly be synonymous with ignorance. To illustrate, a first-grade child might not be interested in a certain kind of food that has a high nutritional value, because he has not had the opportunity to eat it and thus become "interested" in it. Conversely, we could assume that the higher the age level the more we might depend on the criterion of health interest of children. This of course is based on the idea that the older the child the better the understanding he or she should have of needs. Similarly, the older child has had more experience and this is apt to result in a greater range of interest.

SOME BASIC CONSIDERATIONS OF HEALTH NEEDS AS CRITERIA FOR CURRICULUM CONTENT

Basing the selection of health curriculum content on health needs implies essentially that learning experiences are provided in accordance with certain fundamental requirements of children. The use of needs as a criterion for the selection of elementary school curriculum content is not necessarily a recent innovation. In fact it is a matter of record that this procedure was in effect near the turn of the 20th century when the elementary school at the University of Missouri was established in 1904. This school abandoned the conventional curriculum and developed methods of teaching required to make child needs and growth the dominant purpose of the school.

In considering children's needs as a basis for health teaching, certain basic considerations should be taken into account. For one thing it should be recognized that it is not necessarily an easy matter to arrive at entirely satisfactory procedures for discovering children's needs. Moreover, a problem is sometimes posed when attempts are made to determine what the implications of these needs are for curriculum content. In this particular regard, although there is some degree of general agreement that health teaching might well be based on the health needs of children, there is also some difference of opinion with respect to what the needs may be, and what their implications are for the curriculum.

Another important factor is the question as to how much the demands of society should be taken into account as related to the needs of the individual. Various points of view have been expressed in this particular connection. One point of view tends to hold that, because the schools are publicly supported to serve the needs of society, the curriculum content should be based primarily on factors oriented in a direction to meet these societal needs. A second point of view suggests that, inasmuch as it is the purpose of the schools to educate the individual, the curriculum should be based upon the needs of individuals. A rather obvious third point of view involves some sort of happy medium between the first two. This is based on the fact that the individual is a part of society and that he or she should be educated with the idea in mind that there will be interaction with it.

As important as the needs of the child are, these needs should not be considered as separate and unrelated entities as far as the culture is concerned. Certainly, demands of the culture should be taken into account. Such factors as the requirements for social acceptance and the fluid character of American culture might serve as guideposts for proper adjustment between cultural demands and individual needs.

CLASSIFICATIONS OF NEEDS

It is a well-known fact that children's needs have been classified in many ways. However, it should be borne in mind that any classification of human needs is usually an arbitrary one made for a specific purpose. For example, when one speaks of biological needs and psychological needs it should be understood that each of these, although classified separately, are interdependent.

The classifications of needs used here should be thought of in terms of the preceding frame of reference, that is, for the purpose of discussing the use of health needs as a basis for determining what to teach about health.

Two broad classifications of health needs suggested here are (1) those needs that are innate to the individual, and (2) those needs that are based on certain aspects of the environment. It should be remembered that much overlapping is likely to occur in these two broad classifications.

INHERENT NEEDS OF THE INDIVIDUAL

One aspect of inherent health needs involves the basic anatomical structure and the basic physiological function of the human organism. Included here, of course, are the need for food, rest, and activity, proper care of the eyes, ears, and teeth, and the like. Another aspect is concerned with the necessarily of meeting social, intellectual, and emotional needs. This is sometimes expressed in terms of the need for a sense of personal achievement and worth and the need for emotional maturity. It is apparent that an important function of the elementary school is to guide the health learning experiences of children so that these needs may be satisfied in acceptable ways.

NEEDS THAT ARE PRODUCTS OF THE ENVIRONMENT

Many of the health needs in this category might be sub-classified as *immediate* and *prospective* and as   *general* and *specific*. Many of the *immediate* needs are likely to be reflected in the growth and developmental traits and characteristics of children at the various age levels. As such, these are perhaps better classified as innate needs: however, they may also be concerned with some sort of interaction of the environment. *Prospective* needs are those that might be considered in terms of some of the present family and community health problems existing at the adult level. *General* health needs involve those which are reflected in health and safety hazards that prevail on a nationwide basis. On the other hand, *specific* needs might be considered as related to the health status of children in their local or nearby surroundings. As an illustration, general health needs may be indicated from a standpoint of national mortality and morbidity statistics, while specific needs might be determined from sources of information about these statistics at the local or community level, as well as other local information pertaining to the health status of children.

In some cases it might be well to combine the immediate and specific needs and refer to them as *immediate specific* health needs. The following list suggests sources of some of these:

1. Health problems of a local nature that are considered as such by the local board of health
2. Major causes of death in the various age levels at the local level
3. Extent of communicable diseases and infections at the local level
4. Examination of local school medical records
5. Records of local school absenteeism
6. Results of local medical testing
7. Results of local screening tests for vision and hearing
8. Anecdotal records of teachers resulting from observations

PROCEDURES FOR DETERMINING NEEDS

The literature suggests various general ways in which the needs of children might be determined. However, it should be mentioned that the determination of needs of children is a complex and varied problem. An overview of the various conclusions reported could possibly be more confusing than informing. Consequently, it appears important to examine some of the procedures for determining needs and some further approaches and resultant differences in conclusions. Two of these approaches, the *inferential* or *rational* approach and the *quantitative* approach, will be discussed.

The inferential or rational approach, which tends to lack objectivity, is based primarily on reflection of personal experiences with children, and may be subject to the influences of their background interests and purposes. On the other hand ,this approach has the advantage of not being encumbered with possible misinterpretations which may be based on a mass of statistical data. Moreover, it tends to allow for analysis in the light of the broad background, of an expert or groups of experts who have had years of experience in a specific area.

The quantitative approach is found quite frequently in studies involving personal adjustment problems, interests, and other concerns of children. The differences in results obtained usually depend upon the kinds of instruments and research tools employed, and the slanting of statements by individuals making the studies.

Mention has been made that studies of needs may be undertaken by individual persons or groups. This may need clarification with regard to the results obtained. The *statement of needs* formulated by groups may perhaps have some advantages over those by individuals, inasmuch as some of the limitations of individual preparation, past experience, insight, and adjustment might be counteracted by group judgments. However, the value of the statements, whether formulate by a group or an individual, in the final analysis depends upon the abilities of the members of the group or the individual.

The following list of procedures is submitted as a possible guide for determining health needs of the individual.

1. Use an outline of needs to aid in understanding behavior
2. Make use of the results of school medical examinations
3. Analyze personal-adjustment needs
4. Analyze social-adjustment needs

The following procedures may be valuable for determining the needs of the group:

1. Make use of the reports of studies of children
2. Make one's own studies of children
3. Make use of the reports of the studies of the activities and problems of people in the community
4. Make one's own studies of the activities and problems of people in the community
5. Make use of the reports of studies of the activities and problems in our society
6. Explore the ideas of teachers regarding child needs
7. Explore the ideas of children regarding their needs

HOW CLASSROOM TEACHERS CAN DISCOVER IMMEDIATE HEALTH NEEDS

Although teachers may recognize what the general health needs of children are, there still remains the necessity for attempting to meet immediate needs at the local classroom level. This is important from a standpoint of generating child interest in the study of a given health topic.

There are a variety of ways which teachers might use to study particular health needs of children in their own classrooms. The following hypothetical illustration for a third grade is suggestive of such a procedure.

In an elementary school, lunches are served in the school cafeteria, but about three-fourths of the children bring their lunches. These children usually buy cookies, ice cream, or fruit for dessert. A balanced lunch is served, but it has been observed that green vegetables and much of the other food goes into the waste disposal.

A third-grade teacher plans to teach about nutrition in connection with one of the social studies units on *Peoples of the Earth*. However, upon recognizing the situation described she decides to develop a teaching unit on *Foods for Growth*. She hopes to develop the following ideas: (1) that children need to learn why certain foods are valuable to their bodies, (2) that more children should be taking advantage of the school lunch program, (3) that food should not be wasted, and (4) that an interest in eating a variety of foods and of tasting new foods should be developed by children.

The need is apparent to many of the teachers as well as the lunchroom workers. The PTA is so concerned that the supervisor of the lunch program is invited to explain why certain types of lunches are served. A change in the lunchroom personnel, with new methods of food preparation, results in some improvement in the sale of lunches.

The third-grade teacher decides to use a menu for the week as a questionnaire to help determine the needs of her 34 children as far as learnings in the unit on *Foods for Growth* are concerned. The following data are obtained from this questionnaire:

Menu for the Week	Like	Sometimes Eat	Never Eat	Never Tasted
Hamburger on roll	32	–	2	–
Potato salad	23	5	5	1
Orange	34	–	–	–
Milk*	25	8	1	–
Ham sandwich	29	3	2	–
Baked potato	30	3	1	–
Carrot stick	33	–	1	–
Cupcake	34	–	–	–
Baked beans	21	10	3	–
Bread and butter	27	–	7	–
Vegetable soup	23	9	2	–
Toasted cheese sandwich	25	4	3	2
Crackers	32	–	2	–
Jello	33	–	1	–
Fish cakes	5	8	14	7
Buttered beets	6	6	13	9
Cole slaw	25	4	4	1
Peanut butter cookies	20	–	–	14

*18 did not like milk served at school.

On the basis of these results the following questions are formulated:
What foods do most of the children like?
Do you know what these foods do for our bodies?

Do you know why we eat food?

Do you know why we should eat enough of certain foods?

A teacher-child planning session develops, and many worthwhile learning experiences result from the selected learning activities. The latter are based on the questionnaire which the teacher uses as a technique for determining the needs of her class in this particular situation.

BASIC CONSIDERATIONS IN THE USE OF HEALTH INTERESTS IN SELECTING HEALTH CURRICULUM CONTENT

It is important that the teacher have an understanding of the meaning of interest as well as an appreciation of how interest functions as an adjunct to learning.

For purposes here interest will be considered as it is related to motivation. Usually the child is motivated when discovering what seems to him or her to be a valid reason for becoming involved in a certain learning activity. The most valid reason of course is that the child sees a purpose for learning and derives enjoyment from it. Thus, in simplest terms, interest is concerned with enjoyment. The child must feel that what he or she is doing is important and purposeful. When this occurs, motivation is intrinsic since it comes about naturally as a result of the child's interest in learning.

There are certain fundamental ideas about interest that might serve as guidelines to a better understanding of interest as it is related to the learning process. Some of these follow.

1. Interest can be developed by drawing upon the child's experience and particular abilities.

2. Environment has a great influence on the development of a child's interests.

3. There is a constant change of interest as the child becomes older.

4. The child tends to maintain the interests from which he or she derives satisfaction.

5. Interest can build upon interest; that is, the child's interests can be broadened if we capitalize upon his or her present interests.

6. Interests give very important clues to what children want to learn, a very important factor in considering health interests as a basis for determining health curriculum content.

The fact that child interest is a very important aspect of learning offers evidence that health interests of children should be given serious consideration in determining what to teach about health. Nevertheless, there are certain factors that should be taken into account.

As important as it may be, interest should not be the only foundation for the selecting of health curriculum content. Indeed, there are a number of factors that might seriously militate against its exclusive use as the basis for determining what to teach. For instance, it could b very likely that there might be a lack of interest because of a lack of information. In cases where this situation prevails it will be necessary for teachers to attempt to motivate child interest in some of the health problems of the school and local community. Another factor that should be considered, particularly at the K-3 level, is that interest may be focused on insignificant health problems or those that children might not be able to handle at certain age levels. In addition, it might be difficult to provide suitable learning activities and experiences for children at certain age levels even though these children may have a specific interest in a certain area of health.

As stressed before, the near-ideal situation probably prevails when health needs and health interests are in proper balance, and certainly all persons concerned with determining what to teach should be aware of this. As stated previously, the older the child the greater the emphasis that might be placed on health interests as a basis for selecting health curriculum content.

WAYS TO DETERMINE HEALTH INTERESTS

It is generally known that growing children are interested in the health aspect of their own bodies as well as in some of the various health phenomena in the surrounding environment. However, health interests need to be explored more extensively by various kinds of techniques. The following list with accompanying comments suggest some of these techniques.

1. *Observation of children.* Teachers should be alert to the things that children say and do that might indicate some of their present health interests. Sometimes conversations and discussions with children provide the teacher with clues indicative of health interests. The kinds of questions children ask about various factors that pertain to health can serve as a good guide to their current interests. This technique is of particular value at the early age levels.

From kindergarten through grade two, due to the children's inability to write freely, the most revealing data are likely to be procured through the observation of perceptive teachers as children engage in free play, unstructured play and work activities. Of these activities most helpful are health-related events that arise incidentally (life situations), dramatizations, the many health-related questions and such brief discussions as children are interested in pursuing about health events in and out of school.

2. *Questionnaire and inventories.* This type of inquiry form has been used with varying degrees of success as a means of determining health interests of children. It is a procedure that can be used by the individual teacher as a way of determining the health interests of a particular class, or it can be a satisfactory device for ascertaining a general understanding of the health interests of children in an entire school system.

3. *Free writing and checklists.* This procedure can be very effective when the classroom teacher wishes to discern the health interests of a particular class. Children can be asked to write (free writing) three or more aspects of health that they would be interested in exploring. The results of this free writing of interests may be tabulated and the teacher may use it as necessary.

An important value of the free-writing technique is that it lends itself well to the integration of health and handwriting, as will be seen in the chapter on integrating health and language arts. With young children, who may not yet be proficient in manuscript writing, the technique may be used in a different manner. For example, their health interests can be dictated to the teacher, who in turn writes them on the chalkboard or on an experience chart. This procedure can be used to integrate health and reading when the children read the material as it is placed on the experience chart.

Sometimes the teacher may decide to take the free-writing material, particularly that of children at the 4-6 grade level and compile it into a checklist. The list can then be submitted to children for checking those items that are of greatest interest to them. This procedure helps eliminate having the children resort entirely to recalling items of interest.

4. *Health counseling.* In those elementary schools where there is an organized counseling program, a fine opportunity is available for determining health interests of children. The periodic personal interviews with children by teachers and other counselors are apt to yield many health interests that might not be as accessible through other sources. This is particularly true because the child is contacted on a rather informal basis through this medium. As a consequence, some children might be more likely to feel free to express given health interests in the privacy of a personal interview, especially if the teacher or counselor has the child's confidence. Information in the way of health interests derived by the counselor can be channeled to teachers so that they can make proper use of the results of these individual conferences.

TRAITS AND CHARACTERISTICS OF CHILDREN AS SOURCES OF HEALTH NEEDS AND INTERESTS

An outstanding source of both needs and interests of children is their inherent physical, social, emotional, and intellectual traits and characteristics. (A detailed list of these traits and characteristics is provided in the *Appendix*.) The material that follows is provided as a general guide for teachers to help them provide learning experiences based on the needs and interests of children.

It will be noticed that the traits and characteristics in the *Appendix* are presented in terms of age levels. This procedure seems essential for a more complete understanding of the traits and characteristics of average children at a given grade level. This implies that, during the course of a school year, a child will move from one age level to another. For instance, the child usually starts in kindergarten at approximately five years of age, and at the completion of kindergarten he or she is approaching or has reached the age of six years. Similarly, the first grader is approximately six years at the start, and is approaching or has reached the age of seven years when the school year closes. The following scale is based on the age and grade level assumptions made here.

Grade in School	*Age Level*
Kindergarten	5-6
First Grade	6-7
Second Grade	7-8
Third Grade	8-9
Fourth Grade	9-10
Fifth Grade	10-11
Sixth Grade	11-12

The detailed description of the traits and characteristics given in the *Appendix* includes the age levels five through twelve. In examining the traits and characteristics classroom teachers will no doubt profess greatest interest in those age levels that pertain most specifically to the grade level they are teaching or expect to teach. It is recommended, however, that consideration be given to the age levels that are on either side of the teacher's specific interest. In other words, it seems essential that the teacher have a full understanding of the children at the preceding grade level and knowledge of the changes that will be inherent in traits and characteristics at the following grade level. Ideally, each elementary school classroom teacher should possess a general knowledge of the traits and characteristics of children at all age levels of the elementary school regardless of the specific grade level taught. The teacher is then in a better position to see the development of the elementary school child at a specific grade level as a part of his or her total growth and developmental pattern.

The traits and characteristics of children from ages five through twelve in the *Appendix* have been developed through documentary analysis of a large number of sources that have appeared in the literature in recent years. It should be understood that these traits and characteristics are suggestive of the behavior patterns of the so-called normal child. This implies that if a child does not conform to these traits and characteristics, it should not be interpreted to mean that he or she is seriously deviating from normal. In other words, it should be recognized that each child progresses at his or her own rate and that there will be much overlapping of the traits and characteristics listed for each level. A case in point are the ranges of heights and weights given in the detailed lists. The heights and weights are what might be called a range within a range, and are computed means or averages within large ranges. In other words, children at a given age level could possibly weigh much more or less and be much taller or shorter that the ranges indicate.

This chapter has provided the reader with valid criteria for the *selection* of health curriculum content. The following chapter will be concerned with the *arrangement* of such content.

SUGGESTIONS FOR SUPPLEMENTARY READING

Alexander, P.A., et al, Interrelationships of knowledge, interest and recall: assessing a model of domain learning, *Journal of Educational Psychology*, 87, December 1995, p. 559-75.

Carter, M., Curriculum that matters, *Child Care Information Exchange*, 112, November/December 1996, p. 66-9.

Curriculum for tomorrow (symposium) *NASSP Bulletin*, 80, September 1996, p. 1-25.

Foley, J.D. and McInerey, W., An examination of factors in successful curriculum reform, *Planning & Changing*, 25, Fall/Winter, 1994, p. 130-49.

Henson, K.T., Why curriculum development needs reforming, *Educational Horizons*, 74, Summer 1996, p. 157-62.

Liess, E. and Ritchie, G.V., Using multiple intelligence theory to transform a first-grade health curriculum, *Early Childhood Education Journal*, 23, Winter 1995, p. 71-9.

Lolli, E.M., Creating a concept-based curriculum, *Principal*, 76, September 1996, p. 26-7.

O'Rourke, T.W., A comprehensive school health program to improve health and education, *Education*, 116, Summer 1996, p. 490-4.

Schubert, W.H., Perspectives on four curriculum traditions, *Educational Horizons*, 74, Summer 1996, p. 169-76.

Woody, S.F., Behavior mapping: a tool for identifying priorities for health education curricula and instruction, *Journal of Health Education*, 26, July/August 1995, p. 200-6.

CHAPTER 3

ARRANGEMENT OF HEALTH EDUCATION CURRICULUM CONTENT

There are various facets and ramifications of the elementary school curriculum which in one way or another tend to influence the way in which health learning experiences should be provided. Personnel in the field of school health education are continually seeking the most desirable ways and means of arranging those learning experiences which will favorably influence the health knowledge, attitudes, and practices of children. Obviously, there is no standards set of procedures that satisfactorily meets the needs of all elementary schools, because of the varying conditions existing from one school system to another. Consequently, there are certain basic considerations that should be taken into account, involving an understanding of (1) the general ways of arranging health curriculum content, and (2) the topical arrangement.

GENERAL WAYS OF ARRANGING HEALTH CURRICULUM CONTENT

Over the years one of the more difficult problems involved in curriculum construction in the area of health education is that concerned with the *general* arrangement of learning experiences. In the early days of school health education this involved the arranging of content in one of two ways.

One method is known generally as the *continuous plan* and the other as the *cycle plan*. Theoretically, there is an essential difference between the two plans. The former provides for learning experiences in specific health topical areas at *each* of the grade levels. On the other hand, the latter allows for study of given topical areas at a particular grade within a range of grade levels. Taking the topical area of nutrition as an example, when the continuous plan is used, a sequential order of learning experiences concerning nutrition would be provided at every level from Grades K through 6. In the cycle plan the topic of nutrition would be taken up once during the K-3 level and once during the 4-6 level.

THE CONTINUOUS PLAN

This means of arranging health curriculum content is the one most prevalent in the modern elementary school. Proponents of this plan feel that continuity of learning experiences is assured from one grade level to another. Moreover, it appears likely that the child's present and future health needs can be satisfied best when learning experiences are presented at each stage of development. It is suggested also that retention of health knowledge is more likely to occur when learnings follow in a sequential order from year to year, thus providing for suitable articulation between maturity levels in terms of the child's readiness to learn.

There has been some criticism of the continuous plan on the basis that there is likely to be too much repetition of health content from one grade level to another. However, it is questionable whether or not this can be considered a valid argument against the plan itself. On the other hand, when this condition exists, a part of the fault might be due to a lack of progressive sequence as far as learning experiences in the school's curriculum guide or course of study are concerned. Unquestionably, some repetition of health curriculum content may be unavoidable from grade to grade. When it does occur it need not necessarily be a cause of great concern, because a certain amount of repetition of material is not only justifiable, but may be highly desirable in some cases.

THE CYCLE PLAN

As mentioned, the cycle plan provides for presentation of given health topics at a particular grade level within a range of levels. This plan was probably established originally because of its adaptability for use in small elementary schools.

In general, the factors which would tend to favor the continuous plan would be the same ones that might be suggestive of some of the shortcomings in the cycle plan. For example, some persons feel that gaps in health content left from one grade level to another in the cycle plan would tend to militate against the importance of presenting materials at each age level of the child's development. In defense of the plan it might be said that needless repetition of health content is likely to be avoided when aspects of health topics are presented only four times during the twelve years of elementary and secondary school. Many school systems have reported varying degrees of success with both plans.

TOPICAL ARRANGEMENT

A major consideration in curriculum development for the elementary school is the content for any area of learning. All areas of the curriculum deal with relating the content to the interests, needs, and abilities of the individual. These considerations apply equally well to the arrangement of health curriculum content. The factors influencing the arrangement of health content are similar to those used in other areas: yet by its very nature health teaching is unique and different. Health is personal and is concerned with the state of being of the individual as a dynamic living organism. It is a natural corollary that health content is focused upon the basic needs of the individual as he or she relates to the environment and others relate themselves to the individual.

The arrangement of health curriculum content for the various grade levels should be the joint responsibilities of such key people as experienced classroom teachers, curriculum experts, and specialists in health education, and child growth and development.

Based upon a thorough examination of several elementary school health education programs and a documentary analysis of the most recent health textbook series, certain areas of importance regarding topical arrangement emerge. These are *scope, grade placement, development,* and *sequence.*

SCOPE

In general, the health curriculum content as organized under various areas, can be classified by topics of emphasis. Eleven different ones have been selected (based upon the previously mentioned examination and analysis) to include the scope of the content for children from kindergarten through Grade Six.

The major topics of emphasis at all grade levels center around the three basic needs of the human organism, namely, (1) nutrition, (2) exercise and physical activity, and (3) sleep, rest, and relaxation. The eight other topics of emphasis relate more or less to the human organism as it functions in its environment. These include subjects on (1) the human organism-its structure, function, and care, (2) mental, social, and emotional health, (3) clothing, (4) community health, (5) consumer health, (6) safety education, (7) drug education, and (8) sex education.

GRADE PLACEMENT

On the basis of the present knowledge of the growth processes and the psychology of learning, subject matter should be appropriate to the developmental level of the child and the degree to which one can deal with the concepts. For instance, the emphasis at the K-3 level needs to center around practices that will lead to the formation of good health practices in the *care* of the body: at the 4-6 level the children are mature enough to understand the reasons for good health practices through a study of the structure and function of the body. Other examples could be cited from any are of topical emphasis. In the study of clothing, K-3 level children should have practice in wearing clothes appropriate to the weather; at the 4-6 level the children study clothing in relation to regulation of body temperature.

DEVELOPMENT

For the most part a positive approach should be emphasized in concept development, to the end that children acquire wholesome attitudes toward good health. An approach that capitalizes on the importance of a proper diet as a basic need for the body cells to produce radiant health is much preferred to an approach that might cause a fear of rickets or tooth decay.

In the development of content, consideration should be given to the continuity of learning experiences from one grade to another. Concepts that are introduced in the kindergarten should be extended and made increasingly more difficult at each succeeding grade level. The following example of concept development relates to an understanding of the *daily diet*, and is intended to illustrate this point.

Grade Level	Concepts	Learning Sequence
Kindergarten	We choose a good breakfast	Eating.
Grade 1	To be healthy we need to eat regularly every day.	Regular meals for good health.
Grade 2	Some foods that help us grow strong and healthy are meats, fruits, vegetables, milk and milk products, and bread and cereals.	Foods for good health.
Grade 3	Proper foods give us energy; they build strong muscles, teeth and bones.	Value of food to the body.
Grade 4	The body needs a daily supply of foods from each of the four food groups for good nutrition.	Four food groups.
Grade 5	The cells in our body get their nourishment from the materials in foods called food elements.	Food elements.
Grade 6	The amount of food required daily depends upon how active the person is and the energy used by the body.	Food and body energy.

A considerable amount of integration of concepts is needed so that specific concepts extend, support, and strengthen other concepts at each grade level. Moreover, concepts developed in certain topical areas should be closely related to those in other areas. The following example indicates how certain concepts involving digestion appear also in such other topical areas as exercise, nutrition, mental, social and emotional health, and sleep, rest, and relaxation. (These concepts might be developed at about the fifth-grade level.)

Topical Area	*Concepts Involving Digestion*
Exercise and physical activity	Exercise stimulates and aids *digestion*.
Nutrition	Vitamin B helps steady the nerves and aids in *digestion*.
Mental, social, and emotional health	Control of emotions is important for maintenance of proper bodily function *(digestion)*.
Sleep, rest, and relaxation	Rest aids *digestion*.

SEQUENCE

Thus far, consideration has been given to the scope, grade placement, and development of health curriculum content. Another dimension involves the pattern for the sequence of content from kindergarten to first grade, from first grade to second grade, and so on.

This discussion of sequence of content will deal with the eleven topical areas previously mentioned. The arrangement should be considered representative of what might be developed with children throughout the elementary school level.

NUTRITION

With the emphasis on foods and food selection today, nutrition has become a more challenging subject to teach. Children are constantly bombarded with clever, interesting, thought-provoking television commercials. Nutrition, diets, foods, food costs, and trips to the food market are more and more a part of daily home conversation. Meals themselves are the means of family gatherings; some are a part of a particular social or religious gatherings; and satisfying hunger meets an individual basic need.

The primary purpose of nutrition education is to promote the proper choices of foods with time for discussion of the kinds of foods to select, the sizes of servings suggested for adequate daily intake, and the variety of foods available to provide nutritional daily needs. Strategies used to provide learning experiences in nutrition and health are often designed to stimulate critical thinking. Allowing the child to evaluate his or her own nutritional requirements and compare them with his or her present health behavior may cause change, even the developing of a liking for particular foods before thought to be distasteful. On the other hand, the activity may reinforce a continuation of adequate eating practices established in the home.

In kindergarten the emphasis is upon the practice of starting the day with a good breakfast and eating a good lunch and dinner. Stress in the first grade is on good eating practices and the importance of foods. The second grade content carries the emphasis of the kindergarten and first grade, with the addition of selection and variety of foods. General foods such as meats, fruits and vegetables, milk and milk products, and bread and cereals are introduced. Third-grade content deepens the previous concepts, adds care and handling of food, and introduces the idea of what foods do for the body. At the 4-6 level the subject matter should be much more structured. The four food groups are introduced in the fourth grade; elements of food, in the fifth grade and the body's dependence upon foods, in the sixth grade.

EXERCISE AND PHYSICAL ACTIVITY

Effective health teaching is adapted to the day-by-day experiences of boys and girls. Experiences relating to the child's natural urge to play or exercise the body should include indoor and outdoor activities at home and school, at parks and playgrounds, at the beaches and seashores, and on hikes. Giving the children opportunities to develop the physical and social skills needed for game participation is the responsibility of K-3 teachers. The emphasis at the 4-

6 level should be on *why* the body needs exercise and activity, and *how* it aids growth, development, and bodily functions. Physical education activities appropriate to the growth and developmental level of each child should be an integral part of the health curriculum content.

SLEEP, REST AND RELAXATION

For effective learning, concepts related to sleep, rest, and relaxation can be integrated successfully with other areas of emphasis, such as (1) rest before and after meals, (2) rest and digestion, (3) balance of exercise and rest, (4) rest and body functions, (5) rest in the prevention and cure of diseases, and (6) rest and emotional health. The emphasis at the K-3 level is on the development of practices regarding regular hours for sleep and ways of resting, and relaxing. Fourth-grade children learn about the value of sleep. At the fifth grade level the emphasis is on sleep and *body growth and development*. Sixth-grade content deals with sleep and *bodily function*.

THE HUMAN ORGANISM – ITS STRUCTURE, FUNCTION AND CARE

Health teaching fundamentally is concerned with the basic needs of the body. In the K-3 grades the areas of emphasis consists of (1) establishing routines and practices conducive to the maintenance of good health; (2) understanding the importance of body cleanliness, including clean hair, nails, skin and teeth; (3) learning about growth; and (4) caring for teeth, eyes and ears.

In general, the subject matter for the 4-6 level can be classified under structure and function of the body. The fourth-grade content includes such topics as (1) structure and function of eyes and ears; (2) identification of the framework and organs of the body; (3) control of certain communicable diseases. At the fifth-grade level the various systems of the body can be studied. Other health content areas include (1) structure and function of the skeleton, muscles, nerves, and sense organs; and (2) defense against disease. Sixth-grade concepts center around the interdependence of the systems of the body (circulatory, digestive, nervous, respiratory), and glandular functions. (A question of concern here is whether or not to include a study of such sexually transmitted diseases as AIDS under this topical area. In some instances this is delayed until Grade Six and considered under the topical area of *Sex Education*. In other cases, if it is studied at all, it may be a part of the *Community Health* topical area.

MENTAL, SOCIAL AND EMOTIONAL HEALTH

The human organism is an indivisible unity. One cannot look at any facet of growth and development without observing the interaction and interrelatedness of one facet upon another. How the child feels emotionally affects his or her social, physical and mental health, and conversely how one acts socially is reflected in mental, physical and emotional health. Any discussion of mental, social, and emotional health must be relative to the individual at the particular moment. The effectiveness of this aspect of health weighs heavily upon the teacher and the professional knowledge that he or she brings to the situation. From this point of view, the personal development of each child as a complete unity as a matter of degree in development, as observed in the way the child feels about himself or herself, the way he or she acts toward and with others, how the child learns to understand and control emotions, assumes responsibility, and how proficiencies in academic skills are acquired. All teaching situations, whether during lessons devoted to health or not, should be such that the child has the opportunity to grow and to develop to a higher degree of emotional stability, social adjustment, and mental alertness. In general, such broad concepts as the following might be considered.

1. Environmental and hereditary forces affect the mental, emotional and social health of man.
2. Human behavior is complex, tends to be ordered and patterned, and is adaptable.
3. Interpersonal relationships are enhanced by an understanding of self and others.

4. A basis for sound mental health is an acceptance of self and a recognition and acceptance of one's abilities and limitations.

CLOTHING

From the standpoint of health the study of clothing should be concerned with body comfort and protection, appearance and personality. In kindergarten the children need an awareness that weather influences the kind of clothes they wear. In the first grade practice needs to be established for the care of clothes. Attention should be focused on knowing when to wear play clothes, warm clothes, and/or dry clothes. Second-grade children should assume some responsibility for keeping their own clothes clean and neat and caring for their shoes. In addition, they need to learn the importance of wearing clothes appropriate to the occasion and the weather. Third-grade children are ready to learn about clothes for protection, comfort, and good health. The content for the fourth grade should include the importance of clothing in the regulation of body temperature and in the prevention of illness. The ability to assume more responsibility for the care and selection of clothing becomes more evident among fifth-grade children. Therefore, consideration should be given to the color and material of clothing in relation to grooming and appearance. Consideration at the sixth-grade level centers around clothing as it relates to age, durability, economy, and bodily functions.

COMMUNITY HEALTH

During elementary school experiences the child extends his or her environment from the home to the school and into the community. Thus, the child learns about the importance that the community attaches to the health of its citizens. He or she observes the various services available. The child develops feelings and attitudes toward the importance and responsibility of the community for the health and welfare of its citizens. The kindergarten child needs to learn about the importance of the school nurse. The first-grade child adds other health care givers to the list of professional personnel. The importance of using available health services for a physical examination need to be emphasized in the second grade. The hospital can be introduced as a health service. Third-grade content centers around a study of the services of the health department, with emphasis on the need for immunization. During the fourth grade the children can be introduced to community health through a study of the services rendered by the health officers. Emphasis, too, needs to be placed on the responsibility of the individual in the prevention of illness. The topics for the fifth grade can include health laws, health agencies, Junior Red Cross, and pioneers in public health. At the sixth-grade level, subject matter can include a study of community sanitation, health department services, hospital services, and the results of some of the current medical research.

CONSUMER HEALTH

Health advertising is aimed at influencing the choices required of consumers when making a purchase or health-related decision. Consumers of health products often face a dilemma in the midst of a barrage of advertising by the media and friends who feel they have found the answer to a health need.

The majority of consumers in today's society are probably desirous of maintaining a high standard of health. However, the constant reminders through the mass media aimed at children and adults often distort information sufficiently to suggest easy, quick, unusual results to enhance one's physical, mental or social well-being. Sometimes through fear or ignorance consumers succumb to the apparent miraculous results of a particular product only to find they have been misled.

Research has shown that education is a key for providing sufficient information to enlighten children and adults so that they are not further misled. Surveys indicate that consumers are concerned about fraud and quackery. Children can be developing skills in critical thinking and analyzing television commercials and advertising. These skills should assist them as consumers in the decision-making required for making choices about health products, health services and medical facilities. Following are some examples of broad concepts that could be considered.

1. The selection and utilization of health and health-related products and services affect man's health.
2. Health products, devices and services may be beneficial or harmful to individuals and community members.
3. Differences exist between health products and health services.

SAFETY EDUCATION

Safety-conscious children in a safe environment might sum up the purposes of safety teaching in the elementary school. Generally, speaking, there seems to be complete agreement among authorities in the field of health education that safety is an important and essential facet of elementary education at all grade levels. Safety might well be a functional aspect of health teaching related to the child's ability to assume responsibility for his or her own safety and that of others. In general, the content of safety education can be rather specific and structured, since it involves the well-being of children wherever they find themselves.

In the kindergarten the major emphasis is on safety while en route to and from school. At the first-grade level it is important to stress safety to and from school, safety on the school bus, safety with toys and sharp objects, and safety during fire drills. The safety patrol and policeman are introduced as safety helpers.

Safety practices in the second grade include those from previous levels, plus safety on the bicycle and safety measures with strange animals. The fireman is introduced as a safety helper. Subject matter for the third grade centers around safety and strangers, the use of the sense organs for safety, and seasonal safety. Assuming more responsibility for safety at home and for fire prevention is appropriate for third-grade children.

By the fourth grade emphasis is on doing things the safe way and assuming more responsibility for one's own safety and the safety of others at home, on a picnic, on a hike, or in the water. The lifeguard is introduced as a person concerned with the safety of people around the water. Bicycle clubs provide worthwhile experiences for this age child who is seeking group belongingness. At the fifth-grade level children can be participating members of classroom and/or school safety councils. Since they are now mature enough to go away from home with groups of children under adult supervision, safety in the woods includes concepts based upon a knowledge of poisonous reptiles, such as snakes, and plants, like poison ivy and poison sumac. In the sixth grade the effect of one's feelings and emotions on personal safety can be developed. (Sometimes the topic of *First Aid* is included under this topical area and in other instances some elementary schools provide a separate topic for first aid.)

DRUG EDUCATION

Drug education is concerned with the use of such substances as alcohol, tobacco, cocaine, heroin, and various other potentially harmful drugs. In our modern society there seems to be a trend for children to engage in certain activities earlier in their lives. Thus, it is not surprising to recognize that substance abuse has found its way into some elementary schools.

Recently, when discussing this matter with an elementary school teacher, she related the following anecdote. It seems that one of her fourth-grade boys had acquired the nickname of "Tequila Joe" from some of his classmates. With a little "detective work", it was discovered that Joe had been bringing a small container of this Mexican liquor to school several times a week and enticing his classmates to have a drink during recess. In another incident it was recently discovered that several boys in one school were smoking marijuana-and they were third graders. Granted, these may be isolated cases, but the fact that they are happening at all are matters of very serious concern.

At the elementary school level, drug education has been more effective when the discovery approach is used. Through this approach, children study the historical, physiological, psychological, sociological, medical and legal aspects of drugs at their own level of maturity. Each of these areas is only briefly touched upon but does allow for some of the questions children are asking to be dealt with in this drug-oriented society. The concepts can focus on five major areas: (1) need identification and meeting human needs, (2) perception and values and their influence on behavior, (3) building a realistic self-concept, (4) developing meaningful interpersonal relationships, and (5) decision-making.

While an in-depth study of each of these areas is beyond the maturity level of most elementary school children, even at this early age the need to understand oneself as a valuable, unique person will prepare the basis for decisions and attitudes about the use of drugs to alter mood and behavior.

In some instances elementary schools will rely on out-of-school resources to help with the drug education program. An example is *Drug Abuse Resistance Education* (DARE). Once-a-week sessions may be conducted by a local police officer, ordinarily at the sixth-grade level. Among other important information about drugs, children are cautioned on how to react when offered drugs by others.

SEX EDUCATION

Sex education in American elementary schools, if and when it exists at all, is characterized by widely divergent practices. In most instances what is presented, whether it be at home or in school, is far from adequate in today's society. For example, while studies show that about one third of the parents say they have talked with their eight-to-twelve year-olds about dealing with peer pressure to have sex, about two thirds of children say they want to know more about the subject.

Children find that growing up in the world today is a complicated process. Families find that achieving a healthy and happy home life in the midst of conflicting pressures is a difficult task. Both individual and family development require the best use of the human potential from every family member.

An understanding and acceptance of one's sexuality, all that makes one male or female, is an important key to the personal fulfillment of the individual and is the core of any pattern of family living. Sexuality affects the full scale of human feelings and relationships between father and mother, parents and children, brothers and sisters, boys and girls, but the full potential of human sexuality is not easily reached. One must have factual knowledge, skills in problem-solving and decision-making, an understanding of relationships, and a dedication to values that are self-enhancing.

All this is part of the complex process of human growth and development. If children are to be guided along this path, they will require the combined educational efforts of their homes, their churches, their schools and other agencies that can help them become mature, responsible citizens.

Sex education has to do with the joyous appreciation of living, of oneself as a special person, and of relationships with other people-in families and in school, with one's friends, both everyday and on special occasions. It means learning respect for other persons as human beings, the importance of getting along with each other and each person doing his or her part. It means understanding that all living things grow and reproduce, how mothers and fathers care for their babies, that good health practices make for good health, how the human body functions, what changes to expect as one's own body grows, and that some individuals grow differently or more slowly than others. It means learning to tell the difference between what is helpful and what is harmful to others, how to make responsible decisions about one's own behavior, and how to make the most of one's best capabilities as a human being.

Sex education starts at birth when the family receives the new baby and cares for him or her. Much education in attitudes and values takes place at home-some good, some not so good, long before children come to school. Parents continue to be the most critical educational force as long as children are under their influence. As children grow, more sex education is given by peers both in school and outside the classroom. The classroom provides the more formal setting for guided discussion of whatever content has the approval of parents and teachers. The neighborhood, the community, the church, the social class and culture in which children live all can add their own special dimensions.

The school deals with its part by first developing a sound sequential program that deals with basic understandings appropriate to the early grade levels. These basic understandings serve as a foundation for more complex learning that follow in later grades. This program, unlike a mathematics curriculum, will be more readily accepted if the program is developed by teachers and parent representatives together. It should have the support of the community and be specifically approved by the parents of the children who will be taking it.

To develop such a program, parents and teachers need to know first what children are learning from the variety of sources to which they are exposed, and, secondly, they need to now what children want to know as this leads to effective teaching. Third, they should identify what children may need to know for a good start toward healthy attitudes and behavior in the realm of sex and in the broader sense of human sexuality.

A program should be designed to follow children's interests and to answer their questions rather that to initiate them. This way parents have the opportunity to respond to their children's questions at home.

Sex education at the elementary school level can be a great experience for children, parents and teachers, but it needs to be thoroughly planned, reviewed by a group which is broadly representative of the community, approved by a majority of the parents, and taught by qualified and willing teachers. Such a program can help boys and girls understand themselves, become whole and wholesome individuals, and mark another step toward maturity. Following are some representatives broad concepts that might be considered.

1. Individuals are unique and have certain definitive and shared roles within the family.
2. The perpetuation of man serves to promote man's growth and development and fulfill certain human needs.
3. Reproduction, a capability of most living things, occurs universally and reproductive processes are dignified and purposeful.
4. Human growth and development is unique and often predictable.
5. All living things come from other living things of their own kind.

SUGGESTIONS FOR SUPPLEMENTARY READING

Burchfield, D.W., Teaching all children: four developmentally appropriate curricular and instructional strategies in primary-grade classrooms, *Young Children*, 52, November 1996, p. 4-10.

Ediger, M., Sequence and scope in the curriculum, *Education*, 117, Fall 1996, p. 58-60.

Eldred, M. and Fogarty, B., Five lessons for curriculum reform, *Liberal Education*, 82, Winter 1996, p. 32-7.

Foley, J.D. and McInerney, I., An examination of factors in successful curriculum reforms, *Planning & Changing*, 25, Fall/Winter 1994, p. 130-49.

Foshay, A.W., Will we ever balance the curriculum? *Journal of Curriculum and Supervision*, 12, Fall 1996, p. 88-9.

George, P.S., Arguing integrated curriculum, *The Education Digest*, 62, November 1996, p. 16-21.

Humphrey, J.H., *Elementary School Child Health*, Springfield, IL, Charles C. Thomas Publisher, 1993, p. 42-3, 60-2, 73-5, 116-7.

Paulson, K.J., Curriculum-based measurement: translating research into school-based practice, *Intervention in School and Clinic*, 32, January 1997, p. 162-7.

Slattery, P., Curriculum the key to total education, *Momentum*, 26, August/September 1995, p. 31-3.

VanTassel-Baska, J., The development of talent through curriculum, *Roeper Review*, 18, December 1995, p. 98-102.

CHAPTER 4

TEACHING AND LEARNING APPLIED TO HEALTH EDUCATION

It is important that teachers of elementary school health education have as full an understanding as possible of what is involved in the teaching-learning process. Otherwise, they are certain to perform inefficiently and without the benefit of accumulated knowledge from research in educational psychology or the tested wisdom of experienced teachers.

BASIC CONSIDERATIONS

Taken into account in this section of the chapter are two basic considerations which should be useful in understanding the remainder of the chapter. The first of these has to do with the meanings of particular terms that will be used; and the second will have to do with the basic dynamics of the teaching-learning process: the characteristics of the learner, of the subject matter and of the teacher.

MEANING OF TERMS

Every field has its special jargon and the field of education is certainly no exception. Unfortunately, not only are lay people oftentimes confused by educational terminology, but also people in the education field sometimes fail to communicate effectively because of uncertainty as to just what certain words are supposed to mean. The following should make some meanings reasonably clear and help to differentiate key factors in the teaching-learning process.

TEACHING

It is helpful to think of the teacher as one who creates situations in which learning is likely to occur. One factor in this creation is the continuing sensitive personal involvement of the teacher. The teacher should know when to withdraw so as not to interfere with learning, and also know when to step in to provide guidance, help, direction and supervision of behavior so that individuals will achieve the desire learning goals. It is the job of the teacher to adjust to individual needs, leaving some children alone for the most part to manage their own learning, and helping others considerably. The term *teaching strategies* has reference to the teacher's planning and creating whole sequences of learning experiences to build increasingly complex understandings. Child participation may very well be involved in the creating of learning experiences and the planning of strategies.

Clearly, then, teaching is not simply a matter of imparting information. This is to say that it is the job of the teacher to guide the child's learning rather that to impart a series of facts which may or may not be related or meaningful. Unfortunately, even people who think in terms of problem-solving and creative teaching in other subject areas sometimes tend to view health teaching as a matter of rote memory. To them health education is a matter of memorizing some hard and fast health rules and facts.

LEARNING

The word *learning* is used in many connections. For example, we speak of learning how to walk, how to speak, how to make a living, and how to feel about various things such as failing, aggressiveness, going to school and so forth. However, application of the term here is in reference to the teaching-learning process in the school situation. Still, whatever kind of learning one is concerned with, specialists seem to agree that *it involves some kind of change in behavior.* Obviously, the concern here is with changes in behavior that are brought about by the health teacher-learning which is planned for children and participated in by both child and teacher.

Just what does change in behavior mean? This is an extremely important question in health education because it suggests that, due to the teaching-learning process, the child proceeds promptly to behave in more healthful ways. For example, upon learning about the importance of a varied diet, the child immediately begins to eat such a diet. However, the word behavior can also refer to improved understandings as reflected verbally and in writing. Thus, even though a child cannot always change his or her behavior in terms of performance and actually do what has been learned, he or she can reflect greater understanding in written or spoken verbal behavior. Moreover, the child can reflect it in contrived classroom or other situations where he or she is able to act as though carrying an improved understanding into actual situations such as selecting foods or modifying emotional responses. The mathematics teacher usually does not worry too much about changes in behavior beyond what the child can do on a written test. However, the health teacher is likely to be frustrated when the classroom evaluation indicates that learning and change in behavior have occurred but on the actual performance level children may not be putting this learning into practice.

METHOD

The term *method* refers to an orderly and systematic means of achieving an objective. It is concerned with how to do something in order to achieve desired results. Obviously, if desired results are to be achieved in elementary school health education, the teacher must provide the best possible learning experiences for the children. Teaching methods are the means whereby teachers use all possible ingenuity and resources to provide the crucial learning experiences.

Where do teachers look for suitable methods to employ in their teaching? Traditionally, they have tended to pattern their methods after those of teachers considered to be successful. For example, the question-and-answer technique of the ancient Greek Socrates still serves as a model means of building an argument for a great many teachers today. However, in more recent years there has been a growing tendency to look to educational psychology for information about the learning process in order to utilize methods that have been demonstrated to be most effective. Although following the example of successful teachers is still probably the most common source of teaching methods, as teachers in preparation and in-service training have been exposed to the study of educational psychology, the experimental studies of learning have become increasingly influential as the basis for selecting particular teaching methods.

PRIMARY FACTORS IN THE TEACHING-LEARNING PROCESS

For perspective in any teaching-learning situation, the teacher is wise to begin by taking into account what could be called the basic anatomy of the teaching-learning process; that is, the characteristics of the learner, the characteristics of the subject matter, and the characteristics of the teacher.

CHARACTERISTICS OF THE LEARNER

The learner is likely to be eager to learn with respect to health education because the subject matter has direct application to him or her *now*. Every child is potentially an eager learner when it comes to his or her own health. Unfortunately, however, a number of factors tend to militate against such enthusiasm, and these tend to relate to one's previous experience with the subject. That is, healthful behavior may likely have been presented as a series of things that he or she *must* do. Moreover, their is a very good chance that a child may have been nagged considerably by parents and teachers in their well-intended efforts to persuade him or her to do these things. Also, it is possible that some prospective learners have been dealt with in such a way that their thoughts and feelings were not respected. For example, no matter how much a child may complain that he or she is too hot, adults may make the child bundle up because the calendar says it is winter, not taking into account the fact that it may be a warm day; or they may judge the child's needs by their own, not considering the fact that they are more sedentary and the child is very active. The child may be forced to submit to the unrealistic demands of the adult in the name of his or her health (Go to bed early or you won't grow).

Young children may be required to clean up their plates or their trays at school according to the preconceived notion of the adult as to how much of everything the child should eat. Of course this may be perfectly satisfactory to some children who greatly enjoy eating, but others may find this pure torture. Because of their body builds, activity levels and metabolic demands, some children simply require more food than others. Moreover, many children are very sensitive to the way in which their food is served to them. At certain stages, children may be revolted by the intermixing of foods or juices on a plate, whereas they may find the same food quite attractive if separated or placed in receptacles with dividers.

As a final example, children tend to accept the argument that they need plenty of physical activity because they are intrinsically movement-oriented. However, physical activity may very well have been presented under rather highly competitive circumstances in which a certain percentage of children are likely to be designated losers. In other words, something very positive may have been made something very negative, and therefore will be avoided. Similarly, the reasonable admonishment, "Get plenty of sleep," may bring about negative feelings if the child is required to go to bed at an unreasonably early hour.

In brief, it is necessary for the teacher to take into account the fact that prospective learners are potentially eager to learn about their health, but a certain percentage of them have already acquired negative attitudes which must be overcome before the desired progress is likely to take place.

CHARACTERISTICS OF THE SUBJECT MATTER

Much of the subject matter of health education should be intrinsically interesting to children because it is about them and how they can live in such a way as to enjoy life more. Many teachers who have capitalized upon this intrinsic interest and who have used ingenuity in cultivating it have found this can be a very popular subject. There are some teachers who have easily overcome the reluctance of many children who dislike certain foods by making a game of trying new foods and reporting to the class. In other words, the common pride in insisting that "I only like so and so" has been replaced by taking pride (positive reinforcement) in being an adventuresome eater. Similarly, teachers have helped children enjoy physical activity by helping them realize that the important thing is to enjoy being involved in activities rather than being obsessed with the idea of being one of the best performers or fearing losing, failing or not making a good showing.

CHARACTERISTICS OF THE TEACHER

All subject matter areas have their good and their not-so-good teachers. Whatever qualities of dedication, ability to communicate with young people, and enthusiasm for their subject teachers have, they tend to have had at least some preparation for specific things that they teach. Teachers of health range from good to not-so-good also, but it is likely to be more difficult to be a good teacher in this field than in most. A major reason for this is that most teachers do not receive the benefit of adequate preparation for health teaching. As has been indicated, health is generally considered a simple subject and virtually any teacher is considered competent to teach it. As a result, when people are suddenly assigned to teach health, they are likely to bridle and protest that they have not been prepared to do so. Of course, this is one of the reasons for this book; that is to help prospective and practicing teachers feel more confident about teaching this subject.

Over the years experience has shown that when teachers are helped to see the rewarding effects of good teaching in this area, they tend to view health as being of central importance, no matter what else they teach. In other words, when teachers become familiar with up-to-date knowledge about health, the possible contributions of health education to the quality of life of all people, and suitable methods of teaching it, they tend to become enthusiastic teachers. Enthusiasm is one of the characteristics that we see in health teachers who are properly qualified for the job.

It can be most helpful to teachers to consider the characteristics of the learner, the subject matter and themselves when evaluating the total teaching-learning process in any given situation. The interactions of these characteristics have much to do with the quality of teaching and learning in health education.

SOME PRINCIPLES OF LEARNING APPLIED TO HEALTH EDUCATION

In the past the teacher was assumed to be the sole authority concerning what is best for children. Children were expected to learn regardless of the conditions surrounding the learning situation. Today there is a far greater tendency to base teaching methods upon the findings and interpretations of educational psychology. Educational psychologists have attempted to provide educators with sound principles of learning; principles that can be counted upon to encourage learning with respect to virtually any subject. That is, if prospective teachers were to have good preparation in educational psychology, they would be prepared to teach any school subject successfully by applying these principles of learning. However, experience has shown that teachers tend to need help in applying these principles to specific subject matter areas.

The following are adaptations of principles of learning as they apply to health education. They are intended to provide important guidelines for arranging learning experiences for children, and they suggest how desirable learning can take place when the principles are applied effectively to elementary school health education.

1. *The child's own meaningful goals should guide his or her learning activities.* Modern educators generally agrees that if a desirable learning situation is to exist, there must be learning goals that are worthwhile and meaningful to the child. The teachers knows that certain learning goals in health education are highly worthwhile, but children may not realize this without help from the teacher. With the teacher's help these goals should make sense and be meaningful to children so that they will approach them with readiness and be motivated to learn. Thoughtful teachers have utilized a range of techniques to help children see the personal relevance of various health learning goals. Some teachers have found stories especially useful; others have made a great deal of use of audiovisuals and current events to help children find meaning in particular goals.

Of course, the goals should not be too difficult or too easy for particular children to appreciate or achieve. The teacher's understanding of the characteristics of the particular group of learners is crucial in this regard. Learning abilities, disabilities, community interests and problems, and home circumstances may all play important roles in determining goals and how they are to be presented and pursued.

It is important that the child find and adopt goals as his or her own. These goals should not be perceived as the teacher's goals, but as the child's own. To help children view goals as their own rather than as someone else's being imposed on them, many teachers are careful to involve them in the process of setting up learning goals with respect to particular subjects. Of course, a logical next step is to involve the children in planning activities that are likely to help them achieve their goals. These activities may range from readings to field trips and audiovisuals, but they are goal-directed. For example, in one fifth-grade class discussions of current events and a film served to focus attention on certain ecological problems. Further discussion led to the establishment of several realistic learning goals including detailed knowledge of what children can do about some ecological problems, how they might contribute to public awareness of problems, and what might be done about them.

2. *The child should be given sufficient freedom to create his or her own responses for solving problems in the situation faced.* This principle indicates that problem-solving is a major way of human learning–the way of chief interest to educators–and that children must have sufficient freedom to actually solve problems on their own if they are to learn. Freedom to solve problems implies freedom to make mistakes. One of the tasks of the teacher is to show children how mistakes, if evaluated and corrected, can be major factors in learning. Incidentally, learning that making mistakes is inevitable and even a basic human right can be an important contribution to children's mental health at present and in the future. One of the most common problems of many emotionally disturbed people is that they must do everything perfectly or they will not do it at all. If somewhere along the way if they had learned of their mistake-making rights and possibilities for benefiting from mistakes, they might not have become so anxious about them or so restricted in what they are willing to try to do.

Knowledge of characteristics of the group of prospective learners should always be accompanied by keen awareness of individual differences among group members. Some are far more ready to direct their own problem-solving than others. This necessary awareness poses the problem how accommodation can be made for fast, slow and average learners. Children can be expected to solve problems and be creative if the challenge is appropriate to their ability levels. One effective approach to the possible danger of overchallenging some children and underchallenging others is to establish goals that all of the children can be reasonably be expected to reach, and to establish further goals for those children who reach the primary goals ahead of the others. For example, in the ecology project mentioned earlier some of the faster-moving children went on to do such things as interview community specialists and report their findings back to the class. However, it is to be stressed that all children were, and felt, involved in the project as a group.

3. *Children have health interests and needs; however, they may not see value in some of their health needs without the teachers guidance.* Children may, for some practical reason, be *interested* in learning how to cook; but for lack of background on the subject they may not be aware of a *need* to know how to prepare a balanced diet. Under these circumstances it can be predicted that they will learn to cook relatively easily. However, unless the teacher succeeds in arousing interest in the need to eat a balanced diet, learning about balanced diets is likely to move slowly if at all.

Since there is often a discrepancy between what children are interested in and what they need, teachers should consider this entire matter very carefully. Children's interests should be considered carefully because they often point the way to valid needs. For example, in the past, children's interest in play was an enemy to be overcome by the need to learn to work. Now, interest in play is viewed in a favorable light along with learning to work. Indeed, interest in play can open doors to various needed learnings, even in mathematics and reading. In the health field, important necessary learnings may be easily acquired if they are developed within the context of children's interest in play. (Chapter 10 is devoted entirely to this medium of learning.) Thus, imaginative teachers have utilized interest in sports as a means of meeting children's needs for greater knowledge of the benefits of exercise, the importance of a good diet, and the need to work together in a team effort to get things done. Some have even used bans on physical activity when air pollution levels are high as a means of arousing interest in the effects of air pollution on personal health.

In brief, children may or may not be interested in what they need to know. It is the task of the teacher to discover whether there is a discrepancy between the two. If there is, it is the teacher's job to help children develop an interest in what they need to know.

4. *The child should be given the opportunity to share cooperatively in learning experiences with classmates under the guidance of the teacher.* Learning is an individual matter, but it may be facilitated by group interaction, and important social attitudes and skills may be acquired in the process. Learning by means of the group setting can be an important contribution to the overall effort to teach democratic living. For example, in the planning stage of a health lesson children can be taught to appreciate not only the importance of their own contributions, but also to see how their ideas can be improved and expanded upon by the thinking of others. They can learn to contribute to the development of the group planning process. The resulting plans of action have the advantage of belonging to the group and every individual in it, with all that this implies–identification with them and feelings of responsibility for carrying them out satisfactorily. In other words, social skills, like physical skills or problem-solving skills, are not learned at a theoretical level but at a doing or experiential level. Of course, as children mature intellectually they should be taught how theory and practice fit together if either is to be productive.

5. *The teacher needs to provide guidance with respect to the child as a growing and developing organism.* This principle indicates that the teacher should consider learning as an evolving process within the overall developmental process. A principle in the child development field is that *all children grow in their own way and at their own rate.* Individual children rarely grow as the normal curve (that is, a growth curve based on the average growth of a great many children) shows children to grow. Moreover, development is likely to be uneven; physical, social, emotional and intellectual progress do not keep neatly apace. An unusually large child may be slow in emotional-social development, but ahead or behind intellectually; that is, with regard to cognitive learning ability. Finally, in each of the

development areas-physical, social, emotional and intellectual-progress is likely to be uneven. Socialization may be progressing normally, suddenly stop progressing or even regress, and then advance quickly. Progress in learning abilities may follow a similar pattern. The teacher may have no way of knowing how to account for observed changes in individual children. The child's personal biological clock may account for many changes; but deterioration in the environment or enrichment of the environment may account for developmental progress. In any event, the successful teacher is sensitive to all possibilities which may affect learning at school.

An extension of this sensitivity has to do with how much a teacher will try to teach at any given time. Too much intellectualizing by direct instruction may simply be beyond children at a given developmental level. However, a certain amount of such instruction may pave the way to increasing capability in this regard. Thus the teacher must display wisdom as to when to step in and teach and when to step aside to let children feel their own way. In due course, if the material is challenging, it is likely that they will seek out the guidance if not the direct instruction of the teacher.

Serving as a catalyst and facilitator of learning, the teacher watches for indications that children are becoming increasingly capable of self-direction and problem-solving. This is one of the prime objectives of health education; through skillful teaching, individuals who are self-directing with regard to healthful living are created. Making progress toward this objective requires that the teacher be well aware of the developmental process including that aspect concerned with choice-making, problem-solving and self-directing capabilities.

PHASES OF THE TEACHING-LEARNING SITUATION

There are certain fundamental phases involved in almost all health education teaching-learning situations. These phases can be referred to as (1) the introductory phase, (2) the participation phase, and (3) the evaluation phase. No matter what particular subject is to be taught, if the teacher plans carefully with regard to each of these phases, there is a very good chance that teaching will be effective. Obviously, all such planning needs to be in terms of a basic consideration raised earlier in this chapter, namely the characteristics of the learner, of the subject matter and of the teacher. Moreover, all such planning needs to be in relation to the established objectives or goals of the teaching-learning undertaking.

INTRODUCTORY PHASE

The introductory phase provides the opportunity for an overview of what lies ahead, seeing its relevance to the prospective learner and seeing its possible social importance. The introduction may be a relatively easy thing to plan because the teacher knows that most children are eager to learn. For example, the group may be most anxious to learn how to play a particular game and how to build fitness for sports, or learn certain things about human reproduction, or pollution or energy problems which threatens their comfort in winter. On the other hand, some important health topics may not have the advantage of preexisting interest that needs only focusing in the introductory phase. For example, it may never have been brought to the attention of the children that the way they talk to themselves about themselves, has a lot to do with how they feel about themselves, their self-respect and their mental health generally. They may never have considered that the way they talk to others has a lot do to with the quality of their social relationships. Similarly, the subject of safety may seem rather dull, and may even threaten undue restrictions on popular play or adventures. It is the task of the introductory phase to demark the learning area to be confronted, to establish readiness to learn, and to prepare for the participation phase to follow. Hopefully, the introductory phase brings eager learners to the next phase.

Oral and written question and answer sessions may help to establish the starting point of the children's actual knowledge. The group may surprise the teacher with its considerable knowledge or lack of it, and teaching needs to be adjusted accordingly. Testing at this initial stage may also be useful when comparing these results with those obtained later in the evaluation phase for a measure of tangible progress. Going over the test with the class can be a major means of stimulating interest in the subject.

A variety of techniques may be used to introduce the teacher-learning situation. Field trips, stories and current events are among these. Tapes, films and other audiovisuals are prominent among the possibilities. Group discussions and other verbal activities may serve as effective means of follow-up for all such techniques. Such activities can be used to clearly demark the problem, bring out the highlights and encourage critical evaluation.

One of the most important functions of the introductory phase is to establish a continuity of learning from past experience into the present and the future. In other words, what is to be learned is built upon what has been learned before, and it has meaning in relation to ongoing experience. Oral communication between the teacher and the children and among children is doubtless the principle means whereby this continuity is accomplished. Two important implications of this fact are, first, that the teacher needs to emphasize *listening* skills as well as *speaking* skills and, secondly, that nothing can take the place of the teacher in paving the way to learning.

All too often attention is focused on the children's verbal output, their ability to express themselves and the equally important skills of listening are neglected. The result is that people frequently respond to each other, to speeches, and so forth, without having really heard the message of the other person. Of course, this situation makes for pseudocommunication, mostly output and very little input. Thoughtful teachers attempt to combat this problem by emphasizing listening. They call frequently for restatements of what has just been said by the teacher, by other children, in audiovisuals, and the like. The expectations that they are to be held accountable for listening tends to direct the children's attention to the message being presented to them.

Accurate input or getting the message is only part of the process, however, the teacher's indispensable role beyond helping in the acquisition of listening skills is that of helping children find meaning in experiences, including oral and written verbal experiences, is indeed one of the very important functions of the teacher. Each new teaching aid, from textbooks and disk recordings to audiotapes and videotapes and computers has been heralded as a replacement for teachers. But each has found its value as an aid to teachers rather than a substitute for them. If improperly used, the best of teaching aids can be misunderstood or misinterpreted, and their value only part of what it might be. On the other hand, the competent teacher can often use mediocre or even poor aids and, by means of critical analysis with a class, turn them to very good advantage.

So much of human learning is initiated by way of visual and auditory input that successful teachers capitalize fully upon available audiovisual resources as they prepare for new learning experiences. Moreover, they are very much aware of their own role in providing auditory input in such forms as information and instructions. They are also very much aware of their role in teaching communication skills, critical listening and the finding of meaning in what is presented.

Of course, successful teachers also strive for carry over; every effort is made to help children see applications of what they learn in school for other and later life situations where the same skills ad learnings might be applied. For example, critical analysis of a mediocre film at school should help children to analyze television commercials and health-related programs critically at home.

PARTICIPATION PHASE

In the early decades of the 20th century John Dewey popularized the expression that we *learn by doing*. It is in recognition of this fact that arts and crafts courses involve actually making things. Many other subjects lend themselves so obviously to a doing or participation phase that we simply take it for granted. Instruction in passing a ball is always followed by the learner actually doing this. Learning chemistry involves frequent trips to the laboratory to *do* what the teacher and book are talking about, and so it is with many other subjects.

In some subject matter fields there is not such an obvious and established participation phase following the introductory phase. In fields such as social studies, mathematics and history it is more difficult to apply the principle of learning by doing, whereas in biology, children read about seeds growing, plant some and study them as they grow. In physical education they see a stunt demonstrated and then go on the mat and learn the stunt by doing it. Health education is somewhere between these extremes of providing little opportunity to learn by doing and many opportunities to learn by doing.

In some areas of the health field, tying the introductory phase with actual participation (learning by doing) is simple enough. For example, in consumer education it is a simple matter to evaluate products and prices by going to actual stores or by setting up a pretend situation in the classroom for the same purpose. There are many opportunities for creating laboratory situations for learning by doing. On the other hand, some health subjects simply do not lend themselves to laboratory experiences in the school. Direct experience with alcohol and drugs are examples of subjects in the health field which lie entirely outside the laboratory learn-by-doing approach. Learning what takes place has to be at some verbal or visual level of abstraction through words and pictures. Taboo subjects, regardless of their social importance, may not be approached at any level. This is why some of our major problems such as venereal diseases continue to be a major problem. Education and information are not able to confront them at any kind of realistic laboratory level where things are dealt with directly and objectively.

Following are some of the things that successful teachers tend to keep in mind concerning the participation phase of the teaching-learning situation.

1. The class period is planned so as to provide the greatest possible amount of time for worthwhile child participation of some kind.

2. Effort should be rewarded by a reasonable degree of success, and the child needs to *know* immediately that he or she is succeeding. For example, if the child is reading certain material to enable him or her to answer some key questions, both the reading material and the questions must make sense. Then the child should know immediately when he or she has selected the right answers and be corrected when selecting wrong ones.

3. The teacher should always be alert to the fact that young children tire quickly and their attention span is limited. Of course, individuals may vary markedly both with regard to fatigue threshold and attention span, and interest in the subject and its mode of presentation will greatly affect both.

4. The teacher is very actively involved in the participation phase, making decisions as to which children to leave alone, which to help or encourage, and which are in need of special attention. In addition to noting progress with the material under consideration, the teacher is alert to characteristics of the children which affect learning-progress being impeded by excessive distractibility, inability to function successfully in a small group project, or

lack of basic number, letter, color and other skills needed for carrying out the activity. In some cases the teacher is able to provide necessary help and guidance to overcome the difficulty. However, in other cases the child may have emotional, social or learning problems requiring the help of specialists to whom he or she should be referred.

5. In a highly competitive society such as ours there is often a tendency to highlight the work of especially talented individuals and, perhaps to ignore lesser performances. Society needs talented people, and every effort should be made to cultivate talent, especially in areas as important as health. However, such recognition and encouragement must not be at the expense of efforts on the part of the less talented. The competitive spirit needs more balance with the cooperative group spirit. The competent teacher is able to find ways of cultivating talent in the participation activities, while at the same time recognizing and making good use of the efforts of less able individuals. Faster learners are often extremely useful as helpers of slower learners, and by helping them they may well grow in social awareness and in feelings of responsibility for the welfare of others. Such feelings are badly needed in the world today, and no teacher should miss the opportunity to cultivate them.

6. Problems encountered during the participation phase should be noted for evaluation purposes. Are difficulties, problems and mistakes due to faulty preparation or development of the introductory phase? Were the characteristics of the learner, subject matter or teacher misjudged? Were the activity possibilities too limited, not challenging enough, too difficult, not relevant to the interests of the particular group? Of course, one of the most important sources of information on this subject is feedback from the children as well as for the teacher's own evaluation.

EVALUATION PHASE

Except for formal testing to classify children or arrive at school marks, evaluation is undoubtedly the most neglected of the phases of the teaching-learning situation. It seems in most classes (including health education), that when the time allotted to the subject comes to an end, the teaching-learning process ends, no matter where it may be. There tends to be a helter-skelter breaking away from one scheduled period of the day and a plunge into the next. This kind of breaking off tends to be common from elementary school to college, although it is not as prevalent as the elementary school level because the same teacher has the responsibility for teaching virtually all of the subject areas.

The introductory and participation phases of the teaching-learning situation are far more likely to be effective if they receive the benefit of evaluative feedback. That is, just as the navigator of an aircraft is constantly checking its course and either confirming the present heading or correcting it, the successful teacher is constantly evaluating progress toward selected goals and making adjustment as needed. The teacher does not expect inevitable progress toward learning goals without constant checking along the way. Thus, actually, evaluation of some sort is an intrinsic part of the entire teaching-learning process as well as the final step.

As in the other phases of the teaching-learning situation there is ample opportunity for child involvement in evaluation. For example, children can be given the opportunity to discuss (evaluate) the lesson generally and propose ways in which it might be improved. Thus, a problem-solving situation may be created which is guided rather than dominated or directed solely by the teacher. The children are likely to benefit more from the lesson, to feel more personally involved in it, and to find an opportunity to clarify certain points, relationships and applications as well as to grow in capacity to think and talk together in an orderly manner. The teacher may learn a surprising amount about the children, their backgrounds, their knowledge levels, misconceptions and so on. A further value in cooperative evaluation is that all involved are likely to see and appreciate the continuity of lessons. For example, study of obvious pollution problems in the home and neighborhood can lead readily to further study as appropriate of problems in the community, nation and world.

A few minutes of evaluation at the end of each lesson can be of use in determining just what learning took place that day and in pulling things together. This time can help make sure that progress toward major learning goals is indeed taking place. Very importantly, such feedback to the children helps them know how they stand. Recognizing progress in learning tends to reward learning, and it increases chances of further successful effort. Following are some of the kinds of questions which may be raised for brief evaluation. (Of course, the questions raised need to be adjusted to the level of the children.)

1. How can we summarize what we have learned today? Or, have we learned some new things today?
2. Why is it important to know such things about...?
3. How can what we learned be useful to us now? In the future?
4. How can what we learned be useful to others?
5. What else do we need to learn about...?
6. Where can we get more information about...?
7. Are there better ways of learning about this subject than we have thought of so far?

Notice that the approach recommended places considerable responsibility upon children for their own learning as well as their evaluation of it. Also, it gives the teacher the benefit of feedback from children which may be used in the teacher's self-evaluation as a learning facilitator.

RETAINING AND TRANSFERRING LEARNING

Health education is particularly rich in applications to other and later life situations. A high mark or other evaluation on an examination does not necessarily mean that what has been learned in school will be put to use in other and later life situations. How might retention and transfer be encouraged?

Retention of knowledge is encouraged by at least two factors: (1) vividness or timeliness of the learning, and (2) practice. Probably everyone can remember learning things on a single occasion that were retained indefinitely. Such learning may have occurred because the subject or concept was so vividly presented, intentionally or otherwise, that it was unforgettable to the particular child. Moreover, circumstances in a child's private life may make a school experience hit home with special force. For example, illness, injury or a newly handicapped person in the family make teaching at school about home health care, safety in the home and health attitudes toward mental retardation and other handicaps particularly effective and lasting. When the individual's readiness to learn and the presentation of the material coincide, we have what has been called a *teachable moment*. Sometimes teachable moments are predictable and the teacher can therefore prepare for them. For example, whenever children are about to get to do, actually or vicariously, what they are anxious to do, they are likely to be especially teachable in ways that will encourage retention.

Generally speaking, however, the teacher needs to look to *practice* as the most consistently reliable means whereby learning will be retained. Working out means of practicing desirable learnings for retention may be one of the major challenges of health teaching. How might important health concepts be practiced? Some possibilities are: (1) continuing to raise questions about them later, even after considerable periods of time after the initial learning took place, (2) referring back to earlier learnings from ongoing, related material, and (3) rewarding through recognition and praise any evidence that health learning have been retained and even put into practice in school or other and later life situations. Skills of healthful living like other skills ranging from basketball to violin and foreign languages must be used if they are to be retained.

Teaching for transfer is another crucial but often neglected aspect of health teaching. When children learn number skills, do they automatically transfer these to practical applications in other and later life situations- situations like making change, dividing a pie, laying out a play field, keeping score? Perhaps, most do not. Similarly, children tend to need help in understanding applications of what they learn in school to other and later life situations. One of the teacher's major functions is to help children to bridge this gap.

A relatively simple example of bridging the gap is the child's selecting a well-balanced lunch in a play acting situation in the classroom as the teacher helps him or her see the wisdom of making such choices elsewhere, then actually selecting such a lunch in a school or other cafeteria. The teacher can help children see applications beyond the classroom and take learnings into account into other and later life situations.

The basic point about transfer of health learnings is that transfer cannot be assumed. Teachers who appreciate the importance of making application of what is learned in one situation to other situations will make every effort to include teaching for transfer an important dimension of the teaching-learning process.

PLANNING HEALTH EDUCATION LESSONS

Conscientious teachers prepare a lesson plan for each specified period of time to be spent on health education. The lesson plan should take into account all aspects of the teaching-learning situation as it is to occur on that particular occasion. Following are some key points to be included in lesson-planning.

1. List specific learning goals to be achieved during the time allotted. In order to be able to make such a list, the teacher must determine exactly what it is that is to be learned. *What* is to be learned?

2. List item for item, of just how each goal is to be achieved in the next step. *How* is it to be learned? What features of readiness to learn needs to be established at this point? What activities might be engaged in that are likely to encourage learning?

3. Prepare a plan for evaluating *whether* the desired learnings have taken place.

4. The lesson plan includes a listing of desired teaching materials to be used in the lesson.

From the foregoing it may be apparent that the lesson plan is the day-by-day or lesson-by-lesson means whereby the broader health-teaching unit or subject is actually developed. The daily lesson plans become flexible but crucial links in the chain of the total health teaching-learning process.

SUGGESTIONS FOR SUPPLEMENTARY READING

Anderson, J.R., et al., Situated learning and education, *Educational Researcher*, 26, May 1996, p. 5-11.

Brown, A.L., The advancement of learning, *Educational Researcher*, 25, October 1996, p. 37-9.

Foster, W.T., A discovery learning activity to improve student learning, retention and transfer, *The Technology Teacher*, 56, November 1996, p. 34-5.

Lehtinen, E., et al, Long-term development of learning activity: motivational, cognitive and social interaction, *Educational Psychologist*, 30, Winter 1995, p. 21-35.

Pierce, J.W., and McConnell, M., Third graders' use of hierarchies in health class, *Journal of Health Education*, 26, September/October 1995, p. 305-6.

Ross, B.H., Category learning as problem solving, *The Psychology of Learning and Motivation*, 35, October 1996, p. 165-92.

Ross, J.A., Improving student helpfulness in cooperative learning groups, *Journal of Classroom Interaction*, 31, Summer 1996, p. 13-22.

Schroeter, A., Kids learning together: a group for every purpose, *Instructor*, 105, July/August 1995, p. 36-8.

Williams, K.D., Cooperative learning: a new direction, *Education*, 117, Fall 1996, p. 39-42.

Wood, D.N., Learning effectiveness begins with student health, *Education*, 116, Summer 1996, p. 483-533.

CHAPTER 5		

FUNCTION OF THE TEACHER IN THE SENSITIVE HEALTH AREAS

Certain topical areas in health education are considered so controversial that sometimes a teacher is left wondering which is the right direction to take in teaching. This raises the question of how these areas might be dealt with by teachers, and this is the concern of the present chapter.

There are areas in the field of health education that are more sensitive than others. Both illustrate why careful preparation is so urgently needed by those who would teach health. A few examples of less sensitive areas are presented here briefly to show they may give rise to very real problems in effective teaching. They should certainly not be underestimated. However, the chief concern here is with the more sensitive areas, namely alcohol education, drug education, and sex education. These reflect problems, controversies and conflicts within the society at large. They are moral and religious issues to many people, and they are legal and political issues to all. Both less sensitive and more sensitive areas are subject to variations and changes in sensitivity with increased knowledge and understanding of them.

GENERALLY LESS SENSITIVE AREAS

The *less* sensitive areas have to do with certain things beyond the teacher's control which may frustrate hopes of achieving reasonable learning goals. The subject matter may appear innocent enough at first, but in particular situations it may become quite sensitive. The following are examples of some of these. (The pronoun *you* will be used so as to personalize the kind of experience involved.)

You teach a perfectly reasonable unit on nutrition with the basic objective of improving the nutritional status of your children, only to find one or more of the following: (1) your children have no control over their diets, (2) there may be no hope that they will practice what you teach them, for the time being at least, and (3) your teaching violates local traditions. A meat-eating community may react rather violently to your claim that meat is not really essential in the human diet, and that many peoples of the world are very healthy with little or no meat. You may enjoy meat yourself but merely want to make a point that, if one can afford little or no meat, it is good to know that values in various vegetables and other nonmeat products can fill nutritional needs very adequately.

You teach about the known physiological and psychological benefits of exercise, play and sports. Some may protest (perhaps correctly) that air pollution levels are so high that vigorous outdoor physical activity is probably too dangerous to justify on any grounds. Others may protest that education has nothing to do with play or sports, these being detractors from proper, serious education.

You teach that mental health requires flexibility to adjust to changing situations and tolerance of others' views. Mental health specialists may agree wholeheartedly, but your teaching may be suspect because prevailing local standards find their support in racial, political and religious inflexibility and intolerance.

You rightly caution against accepting advertising claims about health products, pointing out that advertisers are in the business of making money, not health education. However, since people are known to be highly influenced by advertising in their buying habits, you may find that you appear, to the children, to be critical of their parents for buying what they do. Then, too, a certain number of parents might possibly be employed by companies that you criticize if you get specific.

If, in addition to some of the foregoing, you give accurate information about deliberate air and water pollution by industries, deliberate selling of unsafe toys, foods, drinks, cars, and so on, or perhaps about political influence of producers of such products, you may be accused of being unpatriotic, antisocial, or even communistic. Your honest effort to improve your children's awareness of health and safety problems which they may help to remedy may make you appear a very negative influence to some.

Thus, if you teach about health and you are at all aware of some of our major health problems, you are likely to have to make some major decisions as to how far you will go in pursuing problems that involve social, economic and political factors.

MORE SENSITIVE AREAS: ALCOHOL EDUCATION, DRUG EDUCATION AND SEX EDUCATION

Alcohol, drug and sex education are not the only more sensitive areas. Cigarette-smoking could be included, but it is not being included here because its established ill effects are too well known. It is hard to find a rational prosmoking argument. Ironically, even the most attractive advertisements are required to bear a warning that cigarettes may be harmful to health.

As mentioned previously, these more sensitive areas that are commonly included in health teaching have certain things in common. Most obviously, society is in a state of psychological conflict over them. While we tend to condemn and reject them, at the same time we are very likely to also prize and accept them. All are the subject of moral and religious conflict. All have important legal and political implications. Moreover, all tend to be more or less closely associated with each other in a *negative* way. That is, delinquent youth and crooked or deviant adults tend to be assumed to drink, take drugs and engage in illicit sexual activities. This is the stereotype, even though many respectable and productive members of society also drink, take various drugs and highly esteem their sex lives. Another important thing that these sensitive areas have in common is an assumed ill effect upon health. However, this assumption is confronted by the fact that each has its advocates who claim beneficial health effects from it. The laws concerning each tend to reflect the general confusion and conflict as well as changing attitude.

ALCOHOL EDUCATION

The enormous sales of alcohol beverages in this country clearly establish the social acceptability of drinking. On the other hand, there is overwhelming evidence that alcohol is implicated in some clearly antisocial and personally damaging behaviors and events of the gravest kinds. These need not be enumerated here because they are too well known, for example, the involvement of drinking in traffic accidents. In Othello, Shakespeare has Iago say, "What is this enemy that men put in their mouths that steals away their brains?" He thereby summarizes the irrational, often damaging behavior that we all know can be associated with heavy drinking. (Heavy may mean two beers for one person and twenty for another.)

In years past, educators were expected to condemn drinking and teach against it. In fact the schools got into the alcohol education business, as they later did drug education and sex education, because parents and others requested help in eliminating undesired behavior in young people. Actually, the forerunners of our modern health education courses centered around the evils of alcohol and narcotics, and this was brought about many decades ago by legislation in some states. However, it eventually became evident that this was an unrealistic approach just as it would be to teach unequivocally for it. The extreme antidrink position tended to force the child to choose between the teacher and much the rest of society he or she lived in, including highly respected parents. Of course, antialcohol education was ineffectual except as it reinforced those children who had already received this same indoctrination at home. Perhaps worst of all, it made the teacher seem irrelevant and out of touch with life.

Finally, impressed by the lack of evidence that antialcohol education was getting anywhere, the schools moved toward teaching for knowledge of the facts and issues, for personal choice as to whether to drink, for moderation if one chose to drink, and against alcohol abuse. (It should be noted in passing that, for obvious reasons, the alcoholic beverages industry encouraged this development with some vigor.) Thus, alcohol education came to qualify as an objective, educational discipline rather than an emotional preachment. As with other subject areas, alcohol education has had the benefit of high-level conferences with expert advice, policies as to reasonable objectives to be sought, development of curriculum guides, and information and support from communities. Thus, those schools that provide alcohol education as a legitimate subject area have gone about as far as they can hope to go in controlling the use of alcohol in society by appealing to individual choice among the young.

To state that schools have gone about as far as they can hope to go under the circumstances is not to underestimate the possible role of the teacher in preventing or reducing self-damaging or antisocial behavior among the young, nor is it to underestimate the possible contribution of teachers to the growth of public awareness of the gravity of alcohol abuse problems. Only such awareness will eventually bring about the social controls and regulations needed to back up educational efforts. As a comparison, good driver education qualified people to subject to the socially imposed controls and regulations of traffic. The best of driver education would not be likely to solve traffic problems if society had few effective traffic laws.

The point is that those who teach in these areas where society is so ambivalent in its attitudes, badly need a realistic perspective. They need to be aware of their limitations in solving the overall problem. This will require decisions and action by a society that so far has not been willing to face up to the problem or its possible solutions.

When teaching in this area that is the teacher to do? Following are some suggested possibilities.

1. Learn from those who have worked before you. Find out what has already been done in alcohol education in the local schools and at the state level. The teacher may discover that both the state and city or county education levels have already given the matter considerable attention. There may already be well-developed curriculum guides, audiovisuals and other materials available for use.

2. Learn how others have fared in their efforts along these lines. In addition to studying the available literature, attend education association meetings where the subject is discussed with respect to research, problems, policies, status and trends, and laws.

3. Find our through preunit tests, group discussions, film analysis, and the like what children know about and how they perceive the whole subject. Teach accordingly.

4. As necessary, use some less sensitive subject such as nutrition as a model to stay honest with respect to treating alcohol education as a legitimate school subject matter. Are facts and their implications your focal point of concern rather than moralizing or selling your own point of view? Are evaluation criteria realistic in comparison with less potentially-explosive nutrition education? Are you being as objective about this subject as you would be if it were nutrition education? Are you overselling a point of view more than you would protein or carrots? Are you underselling aspects of the subject because of personal likes and dislikes?

5. Consider making use of the P.T.A. as a medium of encouraging *family* alcohol education and public awareness of problems and needs. Guest speakers, films, group discussions and literature may be especially helpful.

6. Utilize community resources such as police, physicians and others who are especially knowledgeable concerning some aspect of the subject.

DRUG EDUCATION

Drug education is definitely a sensitive area of health education, particularly when it is concerned with the widely used illegal drugs including heroin and cocaine. Education about these illegal drugs is the concern of this discussion, for it is about them that the dramatic controversies have raged. However, it should be borne in mind that widespread use of many other drugs is controversial too, even thought they may be used legally. Certainly, tranquilizers and pain relievers are commonly overused; and persuasive cases have been made against popular beverages such as coffee and soft drinks that contain caffeine. Adults, especially parents, often deplore the drug-taking of the young, but they tend to ignore the significant role that their own habits play in training their children to expect miracle effects from drugs.

Whereas in this country drinking alcoholic beverages has enjoyed a long tradition of social acceptability, the drugs under consideration here have not. Federal laws were first enacted in an effort to control smuggling; they were seen primarily as a tax evasion problem, which is why the narcotic division is part of the Treasury Department instead of the Department of Justice. As a result, both the selling and the use of these drugs became moral issues, and states enacted statutes severely punishing possession as well as sales with long jail sentences and fines. Interestingly, efforts to control alcohol have had a similar history. Revenuers (treasury agents) were after tax evaders. But it was alcohol as a moral issue, a family and soul-destroying evil, that led to the prohibition years between World Wars I and II. Franklin Roosevelt ran for President on a platform which included repealing the 18th Amendment of the Constitution, thereby legalizing the sale of properly tax-stamped liquor.

Also, as with alcohol, there has been a curious and confusing tangle of economic, moral, legal and health issues that have tended to be seen mainly as moral and health issues.

In addition, such factors as the recent controversy as to the extent to which marijuana has valid medical usage have complicated the problem. This brings up the complicating factor in the whole drug scene regarding uncertainty concerning effects on health. Some of the substances taken orally or breathed are clearly harmful, such as chloroform, sterno or canned heat and glue. There seems to be general agreement that continuing use of the amphetamines (speed) can have detrimental neurological effects. This is why many are concerned about the common, long-term medical use of amphetamines for the control of children with attention deficit disorder (hyperactivity). Heroin can trigger psychotic episodes in some individuals, is addictive to many, and involve severe withdrawal symptoms in many. No one seems to be making a case for the legalization of such substances for general consumption. On the other hand, some of the psychoactive drugs such as marijuana are sometimes described by experts as probably harmless to some people and not addictive. Glowing reports of beneficial psychological experiences such as expanded visual and auditory perception, improved self-awareness, and the like are by no means lacking. Even opponents of the legalization and free use of marijuana tend to admit that when compared to the effects of alcohol, the drug's effects could be mild both in terms of personal health and social damage. This concession is not just with regard to the obvious considerations such as traffic injuries and fatalities, but in less conspicuous ways such as alcohol's role in the lowered impulse control often associated with behavior such as family brawls, child abuse and child molestation which may never even become known. Yet, opponents claim, it makes no sense to legalize marijuana just because tradition makes alcohol socially acceptable and legal.

In answer to the claim that legalization makes for more satisfactory regulation, the opponents see it as placing society's stamp of approval on the use of marijuana or any other drug.

The foregoing differences in views, that is, economic and political implications, changes in attitudes and uncertainties of knowledge, combine to make drug education a very difficult subject to teach well. Typically, the schools have been called upon to deal with the problem because there seems to be no other way of making contact with the great numbers of young people actually and prospectively exposed to drugs. Many hoped that the schools would so impress most children with the likely ill effects of entering the drug scene that few would do so and, therefore, much of the problem would be solved. The call to the schools for help has resulted in drug education programs for teachers and children to sweep the country. Commercial concerns immediately began turning out literature and audiovisual aids to capitalize upon the sudden enormous demand.

Considering the complexity of the problem and the unrealistic hope of many that teachers would persuade or scare children away from experimenting, it is not surprising that drug education has had various degrees of success.

It seems necessary to raise the question as to how far the schools can hope to go in solving problems of drug abuse. These problems involve the entire society, and their solution would seem to require societal decisions and actions beyond what this one segment of society, the schools, can be expected to accomplish alone.

Yet, the schools undoubtedly have an important role to play in drug education when they provide objective presentation of facts and meaningful evaluations of their implications. This means such things as active discussions in which children are helped to use their cognitive capabilities to make rational decisions on their own. Some of these educational benefits may not be evident until today's school-aged children are adults and parents capable of influencing societal decisions and actions. However, in terms of immediate benefits one has to be impressed by the number of young people who, because of school drug education, have evidently behaved more rationally concerning drugs than they might otherwise have done.

What is the teacher to do in this situation where society itself is so obviously confused and conflicted, but expects the schools to come up with magical solutions to problems that it seems to find unmanageable? The following are some practical possibilities.

1. Find out what efforts have already been made in drug education in your school and community, in the local school system and at the state department of educational level. You may discover, or be told, that your job is to teach what the guide says (this is teaching by prescription so as to avoid controversial material) or, you may have considerable leeway. In either case, you will find out what you have to build on and what resources there are.

2. In addition to intensive reading, attend meetings and conferences concerned with research, educational status and trends, and the laws.

3. Go to your children. Through discussions, evaluations of films and other audiovisuals and literature, find out what knowledge and attitudes these young people have on the subject. This is a starting point.

4. Look at your own objectivity. To what extent are you able to approach this subject with the same objectivity with which you would approach a nonsensitive area? Are you able to change your mind as you learn more?

5. Consider expanding into parent education or at least improved communication with parents through P.T.A. presentations, discussions and literature.

6. Utilize community resources such as police, physicians, lawyers, and so on who have something to contribute. Remember even poor presentations can be the basis of subsequent valuable evaluation by your class.

SEX EDUCATION

Some of the earliest training that middle-class children receive is with regard to their sexuality. The blue or pink clothing selected for them at the beginning is part of this. Soon hands are being pulled or slapped away from genitals as parents frown and otherwise establish the out-of-bounds nature in that part of the body.

In brief, mainly through parents, our society at large has traditionally taught children that, except for male or female designation, sex does not, or at least should not, exist. Genitals are for the dirty business of elimination only and should be touched only when necessary. Sex should not be talked about, and those common, nasty words about sex are bad and not to be used.

Then an interesting thing happens. The child presently becomes aware through listening to what is said at home and by the older brothers or sisters or other children, through watching television and movies, and through looking at popular magazines and advertisements, and of course the Internet, that sex is a major interest and preoccupation of practically everyone. Thus, a further confusion is added. First, the child finds that something so pleasurable and evidently harmless, is, by social definition, bad. The second is that the very teachers and policers of the negative sex attitudes, the parents, are very positively drawn to it.

When teaching about sex education one needs to be aware of the dynamics of this strange situation because it has tremendous implications for teaching in this area.

There is the verbal problem which poses a very real threat. For many teachers, the language barrier is a threat both in terms of effective communication and the possibility of getting into trouble for necessarily using forbidden words in the classroom. In other words, it is a unique problem to have to teach about a subject which has no really acceptable language associated with it. This situation is changing some, but for many people even such Latin medical terms as *penis* and *vagina* are unspeakable in respectable gatherings, especially in school in front of children.

Still another complication in the sex education picture is the fact that a great many children in schools have not grown up in the middle class morality concerning sex. These children may have grown up in crowded conditions where observing various forms of sexual activity in progress was not unusual or something to be upset about. In some cases, girls as well as boys are expected to be sexually active from an early age, even before age twelve. Moreover, the only language of sex known may be what the middle class has been trained to consider vulgar.

The foregoing are some of the factors that the teacher needs to take into account if he or she is to understand the dynamics of what is likely to be involved in school sex education. Society's confusion, psychological conflicts and strong emotions are bound to make themselves felt to some degree in the classroom.

The overall trend of the times seems to be in the direction of greater openness about sex. Accurate information is increasingly available to virtually all who want it. The language taboo is not nearly so strong. Mass media are able to deal directly with many aspects of the subject and, even within families where there was the least talk about sex, there is now oftentimes reasonably comfortable discussions of some aspects of the subject.

Following are some practical suggestions the teacher might consider in dealing with the subject of sex education.

1. Find out what efforts have been made already in sex education in the school and community, in the local school system as a whole, and at the state department of education level. The official city or county guide may tell you exactly what you may teach and what you may not, and this may be quite rigid, leaving little to the individual teacher's judgment. Of course, such a teaching guide has probably been prepared by one or more committees, and has received the approval of the appropriate officials. It is intended to go as far as possible, but by all means to avoid controversy. On the other hand, the teacher may have considerable leeway or no guidelines at all. In such a case, it evidently is assumed that the teacher knows what he or she is doing and will follow some criteria as to what is acceptable and what is not. In any event, evaluating the existing situation will provide information as to what one may build on, and what resources have been successfully utilized in the past.

2. In addition to intensive reading, attend meetings and conferences concerned with research, educational status and trends, laws, and so forth.

3. Learn from the children. Through discussions, evaluations of films and other audiovisuals and literature find out what knowledge and attitudes these young people have on the subject. Within the limitations imposed by any ground rules, teach in terms of the evident needs and interests.

4. Look to your own objectivity. To what extent are you able to approach this subject with the same objectivity you would approach a nonsensitive area? Are you able to change your mind as you learn more? Following this recommendation may not be at all easy. In the area of sex, as in few others, people are prone to use their own taste and preferences as the standard to be followed by others-do what I do, like what I like, or you are abnormal.

5. Consider expanding into parent education or at least improving communication with parents through P.T.S. presentations, discussions and the like. It may be crucial to the sex education program to have parents participate in all stages of the development of the program, including the selection of audiovisuals and topical areas to be covered.

6. Utilize community resources depending upon what subjects are to be dealt with. For example, such people as physicians, clergymen, Planned Parenthood personnel and lawyers may have important contributions to make. Participation in your program may help to enlist such influential citizens as supporters of the program. Investigation may reveal that the community includes additional resources such as museums and other possibilities for field trips.

SOME GENERALIZATIONS

When teaching in any of the very sensitive areas, perhaps especially sex education, the teacher is sometimes confronted with a conflict of his or her own. How can one be loyal to his or her own knowledge and convictions and, at the same time, be loyal to established school policies which may set such restrictions upon what can be taught or dealt with in counseling? The teacher may very well feel obligated to inform children about some of the absurdity of certain laws, go into unsavory political and financial aspects of some problems, raise questions about some traditional moral and religious positions, question the sense of the language barrier, and help children break through that barrier. In some cases, such as informing sexually active girls about birth control to avert very serious problems, the teacher may feel compelled to smuggle the information to the young, even though to do so is clearly outlawed.

One can perhaps sympathize with the urge to yield to the temptation to go beyond what is permitted by established policies and study guides. However, there is still a larger issue to be considered before doing so. The issue is, in effect, when is it justifiable to take the law into one's own hands? Perhaps doing so on occasion will do the cause more harm than good in the long run.

If the teacher favors the idea that educational control should be decentralized, and that parents should have a determining say in the education of their children, he or she can hardly make a practice of taking over responsibilities which, in our system, belong to parents and the community. On the other hand, it is recognized that oftentimes community policies are based on traditional, irrational, uninformed attitudes that have not kept abreast of modern knowledge. Sometimes, as in sex education, school policies actually discourage real progress. Admittedly, it is asking too much for the schools to educate entire communities concerning all problems, and severe sex conflicts will be with us for a long time. Yet, the schools can play an important role in community progress by involving parents in school activities, including those associated with the sensitive areas. When confronted with their children's interests and needs, and with the social implications of improved education in these areas, parents oftentimes become eager learners themselves.

Finally, it should be pointed out that problems related to the sensitive areas often need immediate attention and, if possible, remediation. The schools may be helpful in such efforts even though they cannot solve the basic societal problems underlying these problems. The larger concern of society may well be to realize that its major work lies in the direction of providing the young with a challenging environment, and, with such challenging, varied and exciting programs, there would be little need for or interest in escapist activities. This is not to say that alcohol, drugs and sex would vanish from the scene, but they would merely assume more realistic and balanced, less frantic escapist, obsessive status in a generally interesting life. Life can have so much to offer that is not being offered to our children. Possibly, alcohol, drug and sex problems are necessary by-products of our neglect.

SUGGESTIONS FOR SUPPLEMENTARY READING

Berne, L.A., and Huberman, B.K., Sexuality education: sorting facts from fiction, *Phi Delta Kappa*, 77, November 1995, p. 229-32.

Beyer, C.E., et al, Gender representation in illustrations, text and topic areas in sexuality education curricula, *The Journal of School Health*, 86, December 1996, p. 361-4.

Daley, D., Fact sheet in sexuality education, *SIECUS Report*, 24, August/September 1996, p. 22-4.

Gorman, D.M., Are school-based resistance skill training programs effective in preventing alcohol misuse? *Journal of Alcohol and Drug Education*, 41, Fall 1995, p. 74-98.

Jones, R., More than just no (what works in preventing drug abuse), *The American School Board Journal*, 184, January 1997, p. 30-2.

Lloyd, J., Alcohol and young people: a case for supporting education about alcohol in primary and secondary schools, *Educational Review*, 48, June 1996, p. 153-61.

Loveland-Cherry, C.J., et al., Correlates of alcohol use and misuse in fourth-grade children: psychological, peer, parental, and family factors, *Health Education Quarterly*, 23, November 1996, p. 497-511.

Nelson, K.L., The conflict over sexuality education: interviews with participants on both sides of the debate, 24, *SIECUS Report*, 24, August/September 1996, p. 12-16.

Norland, S., et al., Curricula, competition and conventional bonds: the educational role in drug control, *Journal of Drug Education*, 26, March 1996, p. 231-42.

Riley, R.W., Teachers: a bulwark against drugs, *Teaching Pre-K–8*, 27, November/December 1996, p. 6.

CHAPTER 6

INTEGRATION OF HEALTH AND LANGUAGE ARTS

In our present civilization, the use of spoken and written language constitutes the most effective means of communication known to man. Upon the effective use of language rests heavily the acquisition of world peace, the aspirations of people in a democratic society, and indeed the destiny of mankind.

Not only can language affect the institutions of our present society, it can affect the total health of the individual within that society. Through the use of language, thoughts and feelings are transmitted, and ideas exchanged. This continuing process of transmission and exchange interacts upon the physical, mental, social, and emotional health of the individual. As a result of these daily experiences the individual emerges with feelings, attitudes, and values which influence his or her personal health and the health of others.

Classroom teachers fully realize the impact and significance of language in the lives of children. In many cases they attempt to capitalize upon the many opportunities to integrate the teaching of language skills with the various subject-matter areas of the curriculum. In so doing, it is hoped that this integration will serve the purposes of (1) effective learning of the subject matter, and (2) greater proficiency in the functional use of language skills.

FACETS OF LANGUAGE

The language arts program in the elementary school involves the use of language as an instrument for learning. The child uses language in four ways – *listening, speaking, reading,* and *writing.*

Educational terminology refers to *listening* and *reading* in such descriptive terms as the "receptive" phase, the "impressive" phase, or the "intake" aspect of communication. *Speaking* and *writing* are described as the "expressive" phase, the "impressive" phase, the "productive" phase, or the "out-going" aspect. Thus, language has a dual nature. The child has two means-listening and reading-of receiving the thoughts and feelings of others, and two means-speaking and writing-of expressing his or her own thoughts and feelings *to* others.

Oral language consists of listening and speaking, while written language consists of reading and writing. Listening, speaking, reading and writing are closely related each to the other, and represent a single pattern of interrelated, interdependent skills. This is probably best illustrated by the sequence in which the child usually acquires the language arts.

SEQUENCE OF LANGUAGE DEVELOPMENT

Language development tends to correspond to the child's individual growth patterns and to the quality and quantity of his or her language experiences. For the very young infant listening experiences come first. Later, the child speaks the words he or she hears. Ordinarily, during the first year of school, the child reads the words in sentences which had previously been heard and spoken. A short time later the child writes the words. As an example, an infant listens to the word, *milk.* Later, the word is spoken; when the child goes to school, the word is read and soon he or she writes it.

The order and sequence of language development influence teaching in the elementary school. Teaching in one facet of language arts tends to facilitate and reinforce the development of skills in the three other facets. For instance, while the infant is listening and speaking, the first steps are being taken toward reading and writing. It is conceivable that a child can neither write nor read a sentence composed of words he or she does not speak, or to which he or she has not listened.

This functional relationship between the facets of listening, speaking, reading and writing can be further emphasized through a discussion of each facet and its implications for teaching about health.

HEALTH AND LISTENING

It was indicated in the previous discussion that:

1. Listening is an instrument of communication and learning.
2. Listening is one of the two facets of language for receiving the thoughts and feelings of others.
3. Listening precedes speaking, reading, and writing in the developmental language pattern for most children.
4. Listening skills are interrelated with the other language arts skills.

For most purposes of placing *listening* in its proper perspective as an instrument for health teaching a treatment of each of the above points is given.

1. *Listening is an instrument for communication and learning.* Based upon one's personal observation, it appears rather obvious that listening is the most widely used facet of language. Listening is used by people from infancy to old age. It is used during most waking moments of the day either by direct contact with people or by mass audio-communications, such as television, radio, screen and recordings. People of all races and creeds engage in listening during any hour of the day, any day of the year, and in most situations of life.

Through the ages man has apparently considered listening as an instrument for learning. The history of education records the lecture method as one of the earliest techniques for learning. Listening is used at every level of education in our culture from preschool through the university.

2. *Listening is one of the two facets of language for receiving the thoughts and feelings of others.* The other is reading. In other words, the skills of listening and reading are similar in that both of these procedures are used (1) for securing information, (2) for enjoyment and appreciation, (3) for critical

evaluation, and (4) for specific purposes as an individual or member of a group. Consequently, strengthening skills in listening involves strengthening those of reading, because one tends to complement the other.

Perhaps the most significant difference between listening and reading is one of stimuli. In listening, the stimulus is the spoken word, while in reading it is the written word. It should be noticed, however, that effective listening differs from effective reading because of certain factors in speaking which complicate the situation such as loaded words, intensity, and inflections which influence the listener, as well as the effect of group experiences.

3. *Listening precedes speaking, reading, and writing in the developmental language pattern for most children.* Listening constitutes an essential medium for learning until the child can read. In this regard it should be understood that for effective listening, "telling" is not enough. The listener needs meanings for the language he or she hears. Language grows out of concepts which come from personal experiences. For example, the infant learns through first-hand experiences.

These experiences are acquired through seeing, hearing, tasting, smelling, and feeling. By using these senses, the child involves the nervous system and arrives at a concept which is associated with a particular object. Language begins with the word or label which is attached to that object. Therefore, whenever the word which is attached to the object is spoken, that word has meaning for the child. By way of illustration, the infant sees, smells, hears, tastes, and feels the milk from the bottle. From these firsthand *experiences* a concept is built for which the child has the meaningful word *milk* in his or her vocabulary.

Curriculum offerings in the early grades should be purposely planned to give children numerous firsthand experiences from which to develop concepts, and thus to build a meaningful language vocabulary. As a concrete example, in a health unit on foods, second-grade children may examine and classify foods into groups of fruits, vegetables, meats, and bread and cereals. This experience helps the children to develop concepts concerning the distinguishing of gross characteristics of each food group. In so doing, the words *fruits, vegetables, meats, breads* and *cereals* take on meanings for the individual child. Meaning is *not* found in the word; meaning comes through experiences, for concepts rarely go beyond the child's experience.

Building a meaningful vocabulary does not cease with one firsthand experience. Carrying the above example further, let us say that the next day the child handles many kinds of fruit. From this experience, the child learns about kinds of fruit and differences between citrus fruits and fruits that grow on vines, bushes and so on. Now the child's concept of foods has been broadened and extended, and the term *citrus fruit* is more likely to have meaning.

As has been mentioned previously, merely "telling" does not insure effective listening comprehension. Without firsthand experiences similar to those cited, the words *citrus fruits* could mean little or nothing to a child listening to a teacher reads a story about citrus fruits grown in Florida.

At times teachers, in all good faith, think the children comprehend what is being said, when actually the children may have only a vague idea, and can only "parrot" answers. The teacher who becomes discouraged because children have not remembered what was so hard to teach, might well look to the concepts or meanings which children have for the words being used. The startling fact is that at times the most commonly used words may lack meaning for children.

4. *Listening skills are interrelated with the other skills of communication.* The effective teaching of listening skills could mean better speaking, better reading, and better writing. Just the opportunity to listen perhaps has little to offer from a standpoint of teaching a child to listen effectively. Direct teaching for planned systematic instruction in listening seems imperative if children are to improve in speech, broaden vocabulary, and improve in reading and writing. Rather than involving separate lessons, the teaching of listening tends to be most effective when integrated with the content areas of the curriculum, including health teaching.

LISTENING EXPERIENCES INVOLVING HEALTH

When selecting content from the various subject-matter areas for integration with listening, it is recommended that (1) the material have a high interest appeal to children, (2) the information be of such importance to the children that they seek it, and (3) the use of listening skills appears to be the most effective instrument by which the children can acquire information.

It should be expected that children would tend to listen most attentively to material that has a high interest appeal. Health content by its very nature centers around the child as a living, growing organism; that is, it contains subject matter which would be of basic interest and prime importance to most children. Because of this unique characteristic, it might be said that the subject matter of health has "built-in" motivation–a prerequisite to effective learning through listening. For example, first-grade children want to "grow big." Therefore, it should be expected that they would want to listen with intent to information about their bodies growing. As another example, sixth-grade children seem curious, and at times concerned, about their physical growth and development. They may be aware of the uneven growth of their bodies and want to know what is happening to them and why. Their reasons for attentive listening are real and genuine. In such a case, listening serves as a functional instrument for securing information.

When planning for the teaching of listening skills the teacher might want to take into consideration such questions as:

1. What are the experiences relating to health which direct teaching of listening could be involved?
2. What are the listening skills the children will need to function as intelligent listeners in matters relating to health?
3. How are these skills taught?

Numerous classroom situations lend themselves to the direct teaching of health subject matter and the corresponding listening skills. These experiences involve listening to (1) announcements and directions, (2) conversation, (3) discussion, (4) music-songs, dances, instrumental, (5) poetry, (6) programs and assemblies, (7) reports, and (8) stories which are read or told. Outside of school, elementary school children are involved in many of the above experiences through personal contacts or through the media of movies, radio, recordings, telephone and television.

Listening is more than hearing. Intelligent listening involves thinking or a critical examination of what was actually heard. In planning for the teaching of listening skills, teachers should carefully (1) identify each skill the children will need to use to comprehend the subject matter intelligently, and (2) plan questions to give practice in these skills. However, in the actual teaching of the lesson, some teachers tend to omit bringing the children in on what he or she is trying to do and why; that is, *identifying with the children the skills they use and need* to comprehend what they hear. In other words, a fifth-grade teacher when working with children on listening skills might say: "Boys and girls, our health question for today is, 'Why do some people have naturally curly hair?' I have some information on this question which I will read to you. After we listen, it will be interesting to find out what we have actually heard. So listen carefully.

The teacher reads the selection. Then she begins the discussion with her planned questions to emphasize the development of listening skills.

FACTS

Teacher: What facts did you hear?
   (Children listen for facts and tell what they heard)
Teacher: Yes, we listened for facts. So we can say we used listening skills involving facts. I'll make a list of these skills on the board.

MAIN IDEAS

Teacher: What were the main ideas concerning why some people have naturally curly hair?
   (She writes the children's answers on the board)
Teacher: For what did we listen to get this information.
Child: We listened for main ideas.
Teacher: Yes, I'll add the words *main ideas*, to our list of listening skills.

SUPPORTING IDEAS

Teacher: What were *other ideas* that helped us understand the main ideas?

(Writes the children's answers on the board)

Teacher: We can call these statements, *other ideas* or *supporting ideas*.

(Writes words *supporting ideas* over the children's statements)

Teacher: Then for what did we listen to get this information?

Child: Supporting ideas.

(Writes the words *supporting ideas* under *listening skills*)

SEQUENCE

Teacher: As we look at the sentences on the board, let's number them in the order or *sequence* which the writer used.

(Numbers the statements in the sequence which the children indicate)

Teacher: Which listening skill can we say we used?

Child: Sequence.

OPINION

Teacher: What *opinion* did the writer express?

(Writes the children's answers on the board)

Teacher: How can we distinguish the facts from the opinions?

(It may be that some of the statements listed under facts will now be erased and put under statements of opinion)

Teacher: Which listening skill did we use?

Child: Opinion, and that was a hard one.

(Writes word *opinion* under *listening skills*)

DRAW CONCLUSIONS

Teacher: What *conclusions* can you *draw* from what you have heard?

(Children draw conclusions)

Teacher: Did we have to listen well to be able to draw valid conclusions?

Child: Yes. It is fun to think like this.

Teacher: Then, I'll write the words *draw   conclusions* under our list of *listening skills*.

(Writes words)

Teacher: Are there other questions we need to discuss to understand better what we heard about why some people have naturally curly hair?

(Children assume responsibility for listening)

Teacher: The next time we work on listening skills, let's use the list we made today. It should be that we'll have other skills to add. I'm pleased with how well you listened. You are good thinkers.

The preceding discussion should be considered *one* way to teach listening skills. Resourceful teachers find various ways to help children become aware of what is involved in intelligent listening. For the first lesson, it is suggested that a few skills, possibly three or four, be identified. Certain material lends itself better to concentration on specific skills rather than to the teaching of a variety of skills. For instance, a period on listening could be devoted to facts versus opinions, or to generalizations drawn from insufficient evidence. In health teaching it seems extremely important to assist the child to listen critically, to discern health facts, to discriminate between what is actually heard and what was thought to be heard. These skills are among those needed in situations concerning health outside the classroom. Such a procedure might be employed in discriminating the scientific health information from the emotional appeal sometimes used in advertising products through a medium such as television.

HEALTH AND SPEAKING

Speaking is the oldest art in terms of language communication. Of necessity, the spoken word no doubt came into being long before the written word. Through the ages speech has remained the social or "outgoing" aspect of language. It is a means for integrating the individual and the society in which he or she lives and learns. For an effective speaker, there is a listener. Concurrently, when the speaker and listener exchange ideas the listener becomes the speaker, and the speaker becomes the listener. During discussion and while engaging in conversation, a person assumes a dual role. He or she uses both listening and speaking to learn.

This interrelatedness of speaking and listening has implications for teaching at all levels. The elementary school child, by and large, *speaks* the language he or she hears. In language development, speaking holds an undisputed position. As has been pointed out, speaking is a salient factor of learning in its own right. In addition, speaking is basic to reading and writing. When a child speaks in sentences, he or she is better prepared to read in sentences and to write the language spoken. In this context, speaking takes on significant portions as an area of learning in which children need direct teaching and guidance.

Speaking is the second most commonly used facet of language. Some studies indicate that prior to entering first grade the child has learned to speak somewhere around 2500 words. Throughout the elementary school years the teacher uses various ways to enrich and enlarge the meaningful *speaking* vocabulary of children. Among the most common practices involving language are (1) listening and speaking activities commonly associated with firsthand experiences, (2) reading instruction, and (3) extensive reading by the child independently and "on his own".

Through the study of health, many areas of interest, such as food, exercise, sleep, care, structure, and function of the body, are available in which the child may express his or her thoughts and feelings.

Speaking represents one facet of language for expression. The other facet is writing. As previously stated, the skills of speaking and writing are interrelated. Both of these aspects of expression involve the following:

1. Organization of ideas
2. Choice of words to express meaning precisely, convincingly, and clearly
3. Correct grammatical usage
4. Correct sentence and paragraph structure.

There are certain elements of speaking and writing that are different. The elements of speech which differ from those of writing include articulation, change in stress, enunciation, gesture, pitch, pronunciation, and voice. The elements of writing not contained in speech are those which involve capitalization, format, handwriting, punctuation and spelling.

Successful teachers report that elementary school children profit from "thinking through" and listing their objectives or standards for speaking for the year. For instance, under teacher guidance children might examine the tables of contents and indexes of various English textbooks, skim for information, discuss the previous year's objectives, and organize their own thinking. Sometimes their goals can be stated in question form as follows:

1. Is my voice audible and pleasing?
2. Do I speak clearly and distinctly?
3. Do I stand correctly?
4. Do I use correct English?

This procedure can lead into a discussion of what is involved in giving an oral report. Again, the teacher guides the children in the use of multiple English texts to find out what the authorities say. Since the organization of information for an oral report usually involves writing, time should be spent in finding out how oral and written reports are similar. The common elements of speaking and writing should be listed. Children should then arrive at the conclusion that one way to improve an oral report is to improve the notes or outline, or any way that they record the information. Thus, their generalization involves the functional relationship between speaking and writing. In other words, one way to improve speaking is to improve writing.

HEALTH ACTIVITIES INVOLVING SPEAKING

Many situations pertaining to health teaching provide satisfactory opportunities for various types of expressional activities. Some of these "speaking" experiences include the following:

1. *Discussion, planning, summarizing and/or evaluating*
    Discuss and demonstrate good posture when standing, walking, running, and sitting.

Discuss conditions which cause and spread communicable diseases.

Discuss new and/or unfamiliar foods.

Discuss why we should never accept rides without our parents' permission.

Plan a trip to a health clinic.

Evaluate the effectiveness of a health unit upon practices.

2. *Making announcements and/or explanations*

   The school lunch menus for the week.

   The meeting of the Health Club.

   The decisions made by the Safety Patrol Council.

3. *Giving directions*

   Compose a chart on care of teeth.

   Compose necessary rules for safe use of playground equipment.

4. *Interviewing*

   Talk with the school doctor or health nurse about important health practices.

   Talk with the safety patrol boy or girl about his or her problems.

   Talk with a policeman about the kinds of accidents in the neighborhood.

   Talk with the school cook about important foods.

5. Telephoning

   Call an absent class member on the phone who cannot be visited because he has a communicable disease.

   Call class mothers inviting them to assist with the class luncheon.

6. Presenting an illustrated talk or report

   Things we can do to be healthy.

   Health heroes I admire.

   An example of being a good sport.

7. Participating in a panel discussion

   The meaning of good grooming.

   The need for health inspection of public beaches.

   The importance of health inspection of public eating places.

8. *Conducting a meeting of the health club*

   How to preside.

   How to read minutes.

How to make a motion.

How to conduct a discussion.

9. *Presenting original poems, stories, and limericks on health topics*

10. *Participating in creative dramatics*

Playing role of school nurse.

Playing role of mother at mealtime.

The above health activities involving speaking are merely indications of the many possibilities inherent in health teaching. The resourceful teacher needs only to rely upon his or her own initiative in order to provide purposeful activities.

Speaking represents an area of learning which can contribute to the wholesome development of elementary school children. When planning for learning activities involving speaking, the teacher once again should take into consideration the needs of the children as individuals. For instance, the children who omit endings of words ("running'," "playing'") might possibly profit through choral speaking. The child who has the tendency to ramble on and on might benefit by talking from an outline. The timid children might benefit by talking from an outline. The timid children might lose themselves in creative dramatics. The value of such experiences lies in the desirable behavioral changes in the individual child.

HEALTH AND READING

Reading is generally recognized as a most important medium of learning and, as such, it is a part of all subjects. Some of the more subtle types of learning which could involve reading include discriminating, reasoning, judging, evaluating and problem-solving.

There are significant aspects to language development which involve the process of reading. From the previous discussion at least four generalizations concerning reading can be drawn:

1. Reading is one of the four interrelated aspects of language communication.

2. Through the process of reading, one is able to receive the thoughts and feelings of others.

3. Listening and reading are considered the receptive aspects of language communication

4. For most elementary school children the development of reading ability is dependent upon and related to the ability to listen and to speak.

Reading involves thinking stimulated by written symbols. The little black marks on a white page mean nothing to a child until he or she is taught to get from them the meaning the writer had in mind. A part of this involves a basic sight vocabulary and the ability to sound out words by syllables and individual sounds. These are known as *word-attack skills* and include phonetic analysis (phonics) and structural analysis. Phonic deals with the sound attacked to the letter symbols. The teaching of phonics is important, but it should be kept in mind that the English language is only partially phonetic. For instance:

1. There are 26 letters in the alphabet, each with a letter name-a, b, c, and so on.
2. In speech, the same sound is seldom applied as in reciting the alphabet.
3. It is further complicated by the fact that many letters have several sounds. All the vowels have varying sounds (*a* as in map, mate, ant, care, hearth). Consonant sounds also vary (*c* as cigar, cabinet).
4. Many sounds are represented by as many as a dozen different symbols (*sh* as in she, nation, ascension, sure, leisure).

The word-recognition program includes (1) phonetic analysis: consonant sounds, vowel sounds, and rules; (2) structural analysis: root words, prefixes, suffixes, and principles of syllabification and inflected forms; and (3) semantic analysis: meanings and dictionary skills. These represent aids to word recognition and word calling which the children use to read.

It should be clearly understood that reading is more than merely sounding out words. Reading involves a thinking process which includes many complex skills of comprehension. The story is told of a child who read fluently to his mother from a page in his reader. When he finished his mother asked, "Jimmy tell me about what you have read." Jimmy replied, "I don't know. I wasn't listening." Could he have meant he wasn't thinking? A child must be able to do more than call words. He or she must be able to understand the explicit meaning of words, sentences, paragraphs, and passages. Consider the following examples:

1. "A *young* prince stood at the foot of a hill overlooking a *nearby* town." The skillful teacher does not consider a child a good reader when he or she can read fluently all the words in the above sentence, or answers such factual questions as "Who stood at the *foot* of the hill?"

2. "A soldier *without* arms stood by the door." The teacher does not ask a question which requires only the parroting of facts, such as, "How did the soldier stand?" The questions get at the meaning which the author intended to convey: "What do the words *without arms* mean?" "What other meanings do you know for the word, *arms*?"

These examples should serve to illustrate that sometimes the easiest words to pronounce can cause difficulty in reading comprehension because of their various meanings. A child with word-recognition (word-calling) trouble ordinarily is noticed immediately by both parents and teachers. A child with reading comprehension trouble is seldom or ever noticed except by a skillful teacher.

Building a meaningful vocabulary and developing word-recognition skills are but two of the many comprehension skills needed by children for intelligent reading. The many basal reading series, from the readiness books through the sixth-grade readers, tend to focus attention upon the identification of these numerous comprehensive skills and suggest procedures for teaching each in a developmental program.

In numerous elementary schools the basal reading series constitutes one phase of the total reading program. Among other things, these reading series aim (1) to aid children in acquiring functional skills of comprehension, (2) to help children solve their problems, (3) to give practice in reading for many purposes, and (4) to stimulate interests that lead to other reading materials. Thus, successful teachers at all grade levels are expected to assume responsibilities for providing additional reading experience in many areas and for many purposes. However, it appears that in some cases this phase of the total reading program might have been interpreted to mean that children first *learn to read* and then *read to* learn. This generalization tends to imply a transfer of learning and a one-to-one relationship between reading from a basal reader and a textbook of less, or of comparable difficulty. For the most part, observations of teachers tend to suggest that this statement is true only in part. For instance, no basal reading series could be expected to develop meaningful vocabulary in all of the various subject-matter areas. Each subject has certain concepts peculiar to itself, for instance, nutrition, communicable disease, and calories in health; climate, weather, hemisphere, zones, and natural vegetation in social studies; and so on. Without adequate concepts and word meanings related to the vocabulary that is characteristic of the subject, many of the various comprehension skills could likely lose some of their functional use.

As teachers examine their thinking concerning the most effective ways to teach children to read intelligently in the subject-matter areas, they should perhaps give consideration to some of the following questions:

1. Is it necessary daily to have a reading lesson from a basal reader, and a reading lesson from textbooks in the various subject-matter areas?

2. Can the children learn the reading comprehension skills needed to understand the subject at the same time that they are studying that subject? For instance, is it not economical in terms of time to teach the reading comprehension skills needed to understand the health textbook during the health period?

3. Is it not efficient and effective to teach the reading comprehension skills in a functional situation, that is, a situation such as health, where the children see the need for specific skills in order to get the information they need to solve their problem in the day's lesson?

In other words, the point of emphasis involves *reading to learn*, rather than just learning to read. In the final analysis, reading should be considered an instrument for learning and a facet of language communication, rather than a body of subject matter. In such a context, the basal reading book might well serve to sharpen, and to give practice in, the comprehension skills which children need. Experience has shown that children readily understand why they are reading from a basal reader when the teacher makes such comments as, "Boys and girls when you read from the health books you had some difficulty distinguishing facts from opinions. This is a skill which you will need more and more as you get older. For our reading lesson today, I have selected a story to give more practice in this skill. I think you will enjoy the story." Or, the teacher might say, "In our health lesson yesterday, we read about and discussed safety in the water. I have found a story in our reading book which I think you will enjoy. It is about the rescue of a young child from a lake. Furthermore, this is a good story to give us practice in noting the sequence in which the events happened. Turn to the table of contents in the reader."

From this point of view it should be readily discerned that basal reading books can serve to reinforce and strengthen skills needed by the children. It should be borne clearly in mind that this should not be construed to mean that all comprehension skills are not needed, but rather that the teacher through careful diagnosis comes to know the comprehension reading skills in which children are the least proficient, and as a consequence will concentrate on teaching these skills. The importance of this approach becomes all the more meaningful when it is understood that children tend to become bored when faced with drill or busy work involving skills which they maintain through daily use.

In the previous discussion, listening and reading were developed as the receptive phases of language communication. The interrelatedness of comprehension skills was noted and procedures were suggested for helping children identify certain listening skills needed to comprehend intelligently what was heard.

It should be pointed out that children also profit from identifying the reading comprehension skills needed to read intelligently. For example, the teacher might refer to previous lessons involving listening skills in the following manner.

Teacher: Boys and girls, you recall that when we listened to information about why some people have naturally curly hair, we listed those skills that we used in order to understand what we heard. On your desks you have various reading materials to use in solving today's problem: "What happens when we sleep?" After you finish reading silently, we will do two things. First, we will discuss what we have read, and second, we will list the reading skills we used. (After the silent reading the teacher begins the discussion with planned questions)

RECALL

Teacher: What did you find that would help us answer our own questions or the class question?

(The teacher does not repeat the questions. By phrasing her question in the above manner, she gives practice in the skill of "recall"-a necessary skill of remembering. The teacher listens and guides the discussion)

FACTS

Teacher: Let us list some of the things you have been saying. What *facts* did you find concerning what happens when we sleep?

(Lists the facts on the board)

Teacher: What did you need to do to get this information?

Child: We needed to get the facts.

Teacher: Yes, we read to get the facts. It takes skill to select the facts. I will make a list of these reading skills on the board.

MAIN IDEAS

Teacher: What were the *main ideas?*

(Lists the main ideas on the board)

Teacher: What did you need to do to get this information?

Child: We needed to recognize the main ideas.

(Teacher writes the words *main ideas* on board under *reading skills*)

As the lesson continues the children often become aware that these skills are the same as those previously listed on a chart entitled "Listening Skills". It is not unusual for a child to make statements such as: "These skills are the same." "Does listening help us read better?" "I never knew that reading could help us listen too."

For follow-up experiences, successful teachers report that further practice can be given in reading skills by asking the children to read a given selection and write answers to such questions as:

1. What are the facts?
2. What are the main ideas?
3. What are the supporting ideas?
4. What might be a good title for the third paragraph?
5. What are the opinions stated by the writer?
6. What outcomes would you predict?

If the children are to become intelligent readers, this might serve as one technique to use when assisting the individual child to diagnose the skills needing more practice, if he or she is to get the precise meanings the writer intended to convey.

The point should be made here that the quality of an individual's reading is not to be measured in terms of the degree of mechanical skill that has been attained, but by the quality of personal satisfaction and enrichment that was found in the experience of reading.

Throughout the elementary school years, children read for information to use in answering questions and solving their problems. Effective teaching in health should operate on the premise that children learn *by* solving problems that are real and meaningful to them. Although the elementary school is designed to help children grow in their ability to think critically and to solve problems, problem-solving apparently begins long before the child starts to school. There is probably no "age of reasoning" which a child must obtain before he or she can do problem-solving.

Reasoning ability seems to begin at an early age and to develop gradually with experience and language. It is a continuous process, rather than one occurring at fixed stages. Even before the child can put into words what he or she is thinking, attempts are made to solve problems. It is possible that because of the fact that young children do not ordinarily solve problems in words that many people discredit their reasoning or problem-solving ability. For example the one-year old child, pulling the table cloth toward him to get something, is making an attempt to solve a problem.

The use of language as an effective tool in reasoning and problem-solving is one of the great responsibilities of the elementary school. Language includes the printed letter symbols (reading) as well as the printed number symbols (mathematics). The use of reading for solving health problems needs to be taught.

READING AND THE HEALTH SERIES FOR THE ELEMENTARY SCHOOL

An effective health program offers many types of reading for the elementary school child. The current series of health books provide one important aspect of health teaching. These textbooks are prepared by multiple authors, including authorities in health and child growth and development, as well as specialists in the language arts. From the primer through the sixth-grade books, there is a gradual increase in vocabulary load, as well as an increase in the length and complexity of sentences, and length of story and maturity of health concepts used. The teacher's manual accompanying each text gives suggestions for developing the health concepts, and identifies the reading skills needed to read the material intelligently. The effective use of health textbooks can foster wholesome child development while exercising reading skills.

INDIVIDUALIZED READING

Individualized reading represents another procedure for integrating the teaching of reading skills and health.

Various terminology is used in the literature to describe and define this particular procedure. It may be referred to by such terms as "personalized reading," "extensive reading," and "recreational reading." As the term implies, individualized reading is a developmental approach to reading based upon the specific capacity and needs of the individual child and how he or she learns. The major features include opportunities for children to (1) read independently rather than in groups, (2) read books of their own selection rather than of the teacher's selection, and (3) read at their own rate rather than the rate of the group.

The merits of individualized instruction need no explanation or justification. For the most part, some aspects of individual reading instruction are present in classrooms during the library and literature periods. However, many of the proponents of such reading view it as a primary aspect of the basic reading program, not as subordinate or an adjunct.

The extent to which the individualized reading program is carried on is a matter for the individual teacher. Such a reading program has much to offer which can contribute to the total health of the individual elementary school child.

It has been pointed out that in the wholesome development of children, reading and health are closely integrated. The reading materials which can contribute to the desirable objectives include the basic series of health textbooks and the hundreds of suitable library books. The appropriateness and effectiveness of procedures rests upon the "know-how" of teachers, for the way they teach reflects what they believe and accept as their responsibility for the mental, social, physical, and emotional health of children.

HEALTH AND WRITING

It has been mentioned previously that writing is an expressive phase of language. Almost all children want to write. Prior to starting school many children make an attempt. Usually between the ages of three and four years, the young child makes marks for his or her name on birthday and Christmas cards to relatives and friends. From four to six years of age, the child may try to write his or her name, or copy "thank you" notes which have been dictated to a parent. At an early age children have been know, much to the chagrin of their parents, to write on the walls in order to express themselves. For the most part children enter first grade with a desire to write.

As the child develops and grows in the ability to express thoughts and feelings well, he or she moves from writing one sentence "on his own" to writing many sentences involving length and structure and the organization of ideas into paragraphs. Some of the purposes for which children use writing are:

1. Recording summaries of activities such as news, events, trips, and important learnings.

2. Keeping records, diaries, and notes.
3. Recording directions for experiments.
4. Writing letters, such as invitations, requests, "thank you" and "get well" notes.
5. Making labels, captions, signs and posters.
6. Recording creative expressions in the form stories, poems, riddles, plays and songs.
7. Writing his or her autobiography.

Writing in the elementary school is a developmental process which requires planned, systematic, and sequential guidance. A rather acceptable practice of teaching is one which involves group or cooperative writing followed by the individual child writing "on his own". According to this procedure, in the first grade, and continuing at each grade level, the children as a group compose and dictate cooperative stories or class summaries about common experiences. Frequently the teacher records the stories on charts for the children to read and enjoy. A simulated example of a second-grade cooperative health report for the school newspaper is submitted here as an illustration of this procedure.

OUR BREAKFAST PARTY

Mrs. Martin's second grade had a breakfast party at Brighton School. We had cereal, cocoa, juice, and toast for breakfast. Each child had a job to do. It was fun doing our jobs. Our room mothers helped us. Mrs. Greene our supervisor, and Mrs. Stevens, our principal, ate breakfast with us. We had good manners. We enjoyed our breakfast party.

Merely providing opportunities to write will not necessarily mean that children will improve their writing. Direct guidance is needed from the teacher. For example, while recording the cooperative story for the class, the teacher should work with the children on the skills needed to improve the quality of expression, as well as the mechanics of their work. In such a context, the children are more apt to see the need for punctuation, capitalization, correct spelling, and format, as regards indentation and margins. In this process of group evaluation it is possible for children to use the skills practiced in the other facets of language arts, reflected in such questions as:

1. What is the main idea we expressed in this paragraph?
2. Did we include enough supporting ideas to clarify the main idea we were trying to express?
3. What should be the order (sequence) in which we should list our information?
4. What are the best words we can use to express our ideas precisely and clearly?
5. Have we used correct grammar? (and so on with other skills to be taught?)

It appears that such cooperative efforts in writing serve at least two purposes:

1. To motivate the individual child to express his or her own thoughts and feelings through writing.
2. To foster feelings of adequacy in writing.

Again, as has been emphasized in the other facets of language arts, skills should be considered as means to ends and not necessarily ends in themselves. The important factors to consider are that (1) most all children want to write; and (2) they will perhaps write with originality, creativity, and spontaneity.

From the standpoint of health, writing has therapeutic value for some children. Handwriting involves physical coordination and manipulation. Thus, among other things, handwriting entails the use of muscles and bones of the hand and wrist. For reasons of physical development, *manuscript* writing seems best suited for children at the primary level. In this type of writing all the letters of the alphabet are formed with straight lines and circles or parts of circles. The size of the writing tends to decrease in direct relation to the child's development. Although the research in this area is inconclusive, the trend is to be in favor of manuscript for the beginners. Children who begin their writing experiences with manuscript seem to write more freely; that is, they use a larger number of different words than do children who begin with the *cursive* form. (The latter type requires the joining of letters and involves varying degrees of slanting.) It is also interesting to note that children who begin their school experiences with manuscript seem to spell a larger number of words correctly than do children who begin with cursive writing. As the children develop, cursive writing is introduced.

Learning to write is a highly individualized skill. To serve its purpose as a form of communication, legible hand-writing should be produced with ease and adequate speed. An important aspect is the development of what might be termed a "handwriting consciousness," or the desire to write well so that others may read it easily.

The curriculum area of health offers much material of importance to the individual about how he or she will gain experience in writing. In this regard, the following lists of health-related vocabulary words may be used by the teacher.

GRADE 5 UNIT ON CARE OF THE TEETH

brush	dentine	pulp
cavity	dentist	root
clean	enamel	structures
crown	molars	teeth
decay	permanent	temporary

GRADE 6 UNIT ON NUTRITION

beverage	energy	phosphorus
calcium	fats	protein
cereal	fuel	refrigerator
cocoa	milk	skim milk
coffee	minerals	starch
creamery	napkin	sugar
digestion	pasteurize	vitamin

Lists such as these can be used not only for practice in spelling, but for the improvement of handwriting as well.

SUGGESTIONS FOR SUPPLEMENTARY READING

Galda, L., et al, Sharing lives: Reading, writing, talking, and living in a first-grade classroom, *Language Arts*, p. 334-9, September 1995.

Gambrell, L.B., Creating classroom cultures that foster reading motivation, *The Reading Teacher*, p. 4-25, September 1996.

Hedrick, W.B., and Cunningham, W., The relationship between wide reading and listening comprehension of written language, *Journal of Reading Behavior*, p. 425-38, September 1995.

Jalongo, M.R., Teaching young children to become better listeners, *Young Children*, p. 21-6, January 1996.

Jalongo, M.R., Promoting active listening in the classroom, *Childhood Education*, p. 13-18, Fall 1995.

Jones, E., Children need rich language experiences, *Child Care Information Exchange*, p. 126-42, October 1995.

Knudson, R.E., Writing experiences, attitudes, and achievement of first to sixth graders, *The Journal of Educational Research*, p. 90-7, November/December 1995.

Manning, M.M. and Manning, G.L., Reading and writing in the content areas, *Teaching Pre-K-8*, p. 152-3, September 1995.

Manning, M.M., et al, Development of kindergartners' idea about what is written in a written sentence, *Journal of Research in Childhood Education*, p. 29-36, Fall/Winter 1995.

Taylor, J., How I learned to look at a first-grader's writing progress instead of his deficiencies, *Young Children*, p. 17-20, January 1996.

CHAPTER 7

INTEGRATION OF HEALTH AND MATHEMATICS

Over a long period of years there have been many periods of change in mathematics in schools, and believe it or not, there was a time when mathematics was not even considered a proper subject of study for children. In the very early days of this country the ability to compute was regarded as appropriate for a person doing menial work, but such skill was not viewed as appropriate for the aristocracy. Accordingly, the study of mathematics was not emphasized in the very early schools of America, not even the study of arithmetic.

Although over a period of many years changes in school mathematics programs have been gradual, those changes since the mid-1950s have been rather dramatic. These changes can be viewed as an acceleration of the changes toward more mathematically meaningful instruction that had taken place during the previous two decades, perhaps with a change of focus. Several factors converged to help bring about the "revolution" that occurred.

First of all, mathematics itself had changed, and attempts to unify mathematical concepts led to new basic structures that had not yet been reflected in mathematics instruction below the university level. Another contributing factor was the accumulating information about how children learn, for it was becoming well established that children *could* learn quite complex concepts, often at a younger age. Other factors often cited include the concern that the mathematics curriculum was largely the result of historical development rather than logical development, the increasing need for an understand of mathematics by people in business and industry, and a belief on the part of many people that there was an overemphasis on computational skills.

The elementary school mathematics programs that were developed during the late 1950s and the 1960s focused heavily upon concepts and principles and became immediately known as the *new math*. The content of the programs for elementary school children contained more algebraic ideas and more geometry than had been included in previous years. In addition, such things as relationships between operations were stressed.

When the *new math* was introduced into the American educational system it was probably one of the greatest upheavals in curriculum content and procedures up to that time. It also became the victim of much ridicule by educators and laymen alike. One night club entertainer was prompted to describe the purpose of the *new math* "to get the ideas *rather* than the right answer." One of my own mathematician friends, in comparing the *old math* and the *new math*, inferred that in the *old math* "they knew how to do it but didn't know what they were doing," whereas in the *new math*, "they know what they are doing but don't know how to do it."

HEALTH AND MATHEMATICS

Health and mathematics tend to be closely related in a number of significant respects. Planning for the teaching of health and mathematics involves certain considerations. Some of these include the following:

Health activities provide practical experiences for children to have recurring and varied contacts with the fundamental ideas and processes of mathematics through concrete application.
Mathematics concepts are inherent in numerous health concepts.
Mathematics serves as a suitable "tool" in developing health concepts.

Certain aspects of the child's growth and development depend to some extent upon the joint understandings derived from health and mathematics, which complement each other. The subsequent discussions will be devoted to ways and means of integrating health and mathematics.

HEALTH ACTIVITIES AID IN THE DEVELOPMENT OF MATHEMATICS CONCEPTS AND SKILLS

Mathematics is largely a sequential program of learnings that develops through the growth of mathematics concepts based upon previous learnings. The importance and necessity of the children's acquiring a meaningful mathematics education through the use of their experiences need to be underscored for emphasis. Thus, the classroom teacher, at each grade level, faces the daily necessity of promoting activities which are meaningful, applicable, and of genuine interest to the child. It is perhaps in this respect that health appears to be somewhat unique, because it includes many of the activities in which children express themselves as dynamic human organisms. For this reason, through the medium of health, innumerable activities that can serve to develop mathematics concepts and to improve basic skills may be furnished.

When planning purposeful activities, the kinds of instructional materials and the sequence of their use should receive very careful attention in the mathematics program. Consideration might well be given to materials relating to the various aspects of health which might serve to make the learning of mathematics more meaningful to the children. The following example of a teaching procedure is intended to show how health activities and materials can be used to aid in the development of mathematics concepts and skills.

An Example of Concept Development of the Number 2

(First grade lesson at the lower levels of concept development)
STEP 1. The children learn through real experiences; thus, the children begin the development of mathematics concepts at the "listening" and "speaking" levels of learning.
Teacher: Yesterday we made plans to take a walk. We talked about how we were going to observe the out-of-doors. Who can read these two sentences telling what we plan to do when we take our walk this afternoon?
Child: (reads from illustrated chart)
We will look with our two eyes.
We will listen with our two ears.
Teacher: You read well. Now how many eyes will we use?
(Note: The children begin to develop the concepts of: (1) quantity or "how many," and (2) the cardinal number 2.)

Child: Two eyes.

Teacher: Let's point to our two eyes.

    (Children point to their two eyes.)

Teacher: How many ears will we use?

Child: Two ears.

Teacher: Let's point to our two ears.

    (Children point to their two ears.)

Teacher: For our mathematics lesson today, we are going to learn about the number 2, and what it means. We have just pointed to our two eyes and two ears. Let's think about other parts of our body. As we do, I am going to ask you to do two things: first, find two other parts of the body that are alike; second, tell us what the two parts are.

    (Note: The teacher introduces the ordinal numbers, first and second, as a part of the children's "listening" vocabulary.)

Child: I have two feet.

Teacher: Let's point to our two feet and count them – one, two.

    (Note: Children point to their feet as they begin to develop the concept of rational counting.)

Teacher: Who can tell us about two other similar parts of the body?

Child: I have two hands.

Teacher: Let's point to our two hands and count them – one, two.

    (Note: Under teacher guidance the children continue to develop the concepts of quantity and rational counting, as they identify two similar parts of the body.)

Child Responses:

    I have two cheeks – one, two.

    I have two lips – one, two.

    I have two eyebrows – one, two.

    I have two shoulders – one, two.

    I have two arms – one, two.

    I have two elbows – one, two.

    I have two wrists – one, two.

    I have two hips – one, two.

    I have two legs – one, two.

    I have two knees – one, two.

    I have two ankles – one, two.

STEP 2. The children manipulate concrete objects involving the play and exercise aspects of health to develop and extend their concepts of the number 2. This activity is presented also at the "listening and speaking" levels.

Teacher: When we go outside for recess this morning we can take turns playing with the different things I have for you on the table. As you come to the table I would like you to do two things: first, select two items that are alike to take outside, second, tell us how you can use them.

(Note: The teacher again presents the ordinal numbers, first and second, as a part of the children's listening vocabulary.)

Child: I have two bean bags. I will throw my two bean bags.

Teacher: To whom will you throw them?

Child: To Billy.

Teacher: If Billy and Jack play with the bean bags, how many children will be playing with them?

Child: Two children.

Teacher: Billy and Jack, please stand so we can count you.

Children: One, two.

Teacher: Then for two things to play with we need two children. We are finding many ways to use the number 2.

(Note: Under teacher guidance, the children use the number 2 in their "speaking" vocabulary, as they manipulate the concrete objects. The building of a number vocabulary – little, big, short, long – proceeds concurrently with the development of the number concept.)

Child Responses:

I have two jump ropes.

Two of us can jump rope.

I have two long jump ropes.

Two of us can hold each rope.

Two children can jump the two ropes.

I have two wooden blocks.

Two of us can make up a game to play with them.

Teacher: You may put the things that you will play with under your chairs until it is time for recess.

STEP 3. The children use semiconcrete objects (pictures) to extend their concepts of the number.

Teacher: On the chalkboard ledge there are colored pictures of things to eat. You may keep the pictures you select to paste in your own mathematics scrapbook. As you come up I would like you to do two things: first, select two items of food that are alike, and second, tell us in a sentence what you have selected as you count the items.

(Note: Again the teacher presents the ordinal numbers, first and second, as a part of the "listening" vocabulary.)

Child: I have two apples – one, two.

(Note: Under teacher guidance at this level of concept development the children use the number 2 to identify semiconcrete objects.)

Child Responses:

I have two oranges – one, two.

I have two pears – one, two.

I have two carrots – one, two.

I have two potatoes – one, two.

Teacher: We have used the number 2 to talk about many things this morning.

What are some of the ways we used the number 2?

(Note: The teacher helps the children to arrive at generalizations, such as, "The number two can be used to mean two people, two parts of the body, two playthings, two foods, and other things too. The number 2 can be used to count.")

Teacher: Did you realize that so many things come in twos?

Tomorrow we are going to learn even more about number 2.

Teacher: It is now snack time. Today as usual you will be served milk and how many cookies?

Child: Two cookies.

STEP 4. This usually involves the use of the abstract symbol in the "reading and writing" stage of development (2-two). The use of the mathematics textbook can be introduced at this point for additional information and practice.

While reinforcing these concepts, other ideas will be introduced to extend the meanings in the growth of mathematics concepts associated with the number symbol 2, at the early level, as well as at all higher levels. As illustrated in the preceding lesson the resourceful teacher can then turn to health for many meaningful activities to develop and extend such concepts as:

1. Cardinal aspects of quantity and grouping, including the ability to associate a quantity with the corresponding number symbol.

Example: Two dots (..) can be associated with the umber symbol 2.

2. Ordinal or "place in a series" aspect of number.

Example: Jack is first; Mary is second.

3. Rote counting in sequence involving learning to speak, read, and write the symbol and corresponding number name.

Example: Counting in sequence by saying, "1, 2, 3," and so on. Knowing which number comes before 2 (sequence). Knowing which number comes after 2 (sequence). Writing the number symbol and corresponding number name - 2, two.

4. Rational counting involving one-to-one relationship.

Example: Pointing to an object such as an apple and saying "one," Pointing to the next apple and saying "two", and so on.

5. Development of a meaningful mathematics vocabulary involving the number two, such as:

Number words: two, twice, pair, half, second, and so on.

Example: Two is twice as big as 1, or 2:1 (ratio). Two is one-half of 4, or 2/4=1/2 or 4 divided by 2=2. "I have a pair of gloves." "I sit in the second seat."

Placement "two" can have many positions left and right of the decimal.

Example: 2 tenths of 1 is 0.2 2 hundredths of 1 is .02.

2 ones or 2. 2 tens or 20. 2 hundreds or 200. 2 thousands or 2000.

Inequality of numbers: more than, less than, the same as, and so on.

Example: 2 is more than 1. 2 is less than 3. 1 and 1 are usually the same as 2 and 0.

Measurements: area, time, temperature, and the like, using the number 2.

Example: temperature (72 degrees)-room. weight (2 ounces, 2 pounds, and so on)-foods. liquid measures (2 cups, 2 pints, and so on)-milk, water. linear dimensions (2 inches, 2 feet, and so on)-clothing. area (2 sq. inches, 2 sq. feet)-play and safety areas. time (2 seconds, 2 minutes, 2 hours, and so on)-sleep, rest. money (2 coins, 2 cents, 2 nickels, and so on)-cost of foods.

6. Mathematics concepts that spiral to higher levels.

Commutative Law: The order in which numbers are added does not affect the sum.

Example: 2 and 1 are 1 and 2.

$1 + 2 = 2 + 1$.

$1 + 0 + 2 = 2 + 1 + 0$

Commutative Law: The order in which numbers are multiplied does not affect the product.

Example: $2 \times 1 = 1 \times 2$

2   1

X1 X2

2   2

Associative Law: The order in which numbers are grouped does not affect the sum.

Example: $1 + (1+0)=(0+1)+1$

Associative Law: The order in which numbers are grouped does not affect the product

Example: $(1x0)x2=1(0x2)$

Distributive Law: To multiply an indicated sum by a number, each addend must be multiplied by that number.

Example: $2(1+0)=(2x1)+(2x0)$

Identity Law of Addition: Adding zero to a number does not change the number.

$2 + 0 = 2$

Two and zero are two.

Identity Law of Multiplication: Multiplying a number by 1 does not change the number.

Example: $1 x 2 = 2$

7. Two dimensions of a plane. Illustrations are limited for the most part to two dimensions.

8. Square root. In finding a square root, 2 is the index of radical.

9. Equations. An equation is an algebraic expression in which two quantities under certain conditions are equal.

10. Base of the binary system. The binary system uses 2 as a base. The binary system is used extensively in present-day high-speed computational machines.

The sequence of materials used in the preceding example follows a rather structured pattern: step one, use of real experiences; step 2, use of concrete objects; step 3, use of semiconcrete objects; step 4, use of the abstract symbol. Steps 1 and 2 are at a low concept level and the experiences are at the "listening and speaking" stage of development. Step 4, using abstractions is a the "reading and writing" stage of development. Mathematics concepts started at the lowest level, as in the above example of the number 2, can continuously be expanded into more complex and difficult mathematics ideas.

It is hoped that the preceding discussion has served to identify a few of the numerous aspects of health, such as body parts, play and exercise activities, and foods, which could be used to give practice in basic number skills, as well as to develop and extend mathematics concepts.

DEVELOPMENT OF MATHEMATICS CONCEPTS AND HEALTH CONCEPTS

Health activities can provide meaningful experiences to aid in the development of health concepts. In addition, health teaching, to accomplish its total objectives, must rely to a certain extent upon the effective use of mathematics concepts and skills. From this point of view, the obvious necessity for integration of health and mathematics takes on added significance.

In many cases numerous mathematics concepts are inherent in health concepts. When the teacher is aware of this it is very likely that a better development of *both* types of concepts will accrue.

In mathematics teaching, as in health, it is essential that basic mathematics concepts be developed and extended continuously through the entire mathematics curriculum from kindergarten through college. Thus, no one concept can be said to begin or end at any particular level of one's education.

An examination of the concepts listed below should serve to illustrate some of the mathematics concepts that are inherent in health teaching at the grade levels K-6.

Health Concepts   *Inherent Mathematics Concepts*

Grades K-3

Health Concepts	Inherent Mathematics Concepts
We drink water every day.	Liquid measurements.
Regular hours for going to bed and for getting up help us get the sleep we need.	Time involving minutes, hours, days of week.
We grow during the night as well as during the day. When weighed and measured regularly, we can check on how much we are growing	Measurement of time, weight, length.
Milk helps us grow strong and healthy	Vocabulary including "how much;" liquid measurement.
Some foods that help us grow strong and healthy are meats, fruits and vegetables, milk and milk products, bread and cereals.	Grouping, counting, addition, measurements.

When we walk, stand and sit correctly we help ourselves grow. Height and weight are measures of growth. Each boy and girl grows in his or her own way.	Measurements of height, length, time.
A regular amount of sleep each night can make us lively and happy. We have five senses that help us know about and enjoy life.	Time, involving minutes, hours, days of the week. Rational counting, grouping.

Grades 4-6

There are four groups of foods important to good health Sufficient sleep aids growth.	Grouping, circle graphs, pyramid graphs. Measurements of time in whole numbers and fractions.
Clothes help us maintain normal temperature.	Reading and writing numbers on thermometers; decimals.
Changes in size are an important aspect of physical growth; we grow at different rates, in different ways, at different times.	Measurements, averages, fractions.
We have four kinds of teeth, each useful in a different way.	Addition, grouping, division involving partition.
We can help to care for our eyes by sitting a proper distance from a television or movie screen.	Measurements of length.
Vibrations of the vocal chords in the larynx make us able to speak.	Comparison of frequencies of different sound waves; comparison of speed of light to speed of sound. Use of decimal fractions.
When we are well, our temperature remains at approximately 98.6 degrees.	
Our framework consists of the head, neck, trunk, arms, and legs; the trunk consists of the chest and abdomen, which contain vital organs.	Counting, grouping, addition with carrying.
We are made up of millions of living cells which require food to grow, to repair themselves, and to produce energy and heat.	Multiples of millions, relationship of millions of cells to thousands, hundreds, and tens of cells.

The smallest part of us is a cell; we grow because cells divide to make new cells.	Comparison of sizes; fractions; multiplication.
The pituitary gland, located at the base of the brain, regulates our growth in height.	Measurement of growth.
Individual differences in height, weight, and build among children of the same age are to be expected.	Comparisons of size; relationships of length of arm spread to height.
Our brain is made up of millions of nerve cells.	Multiples of millions; relationship of millions of cells to billions and trillions of cells.
Since no single food contains all essentials, our cells require a supply of the four basic elements daily.	Comparison of caloric count in foods; addition of caloric count of foods in daily diet; averaging of calories.
Physical activity increases the respiration rate and the rate of the heart.	Averaging rates; comparison of respiration rate and rate of heartbeat.
A change in air pressure causes a new sensation in the ear due to changes in pressure on the eardrum.	Recording of air pressure; measurement of volume.

MATHEMATICS AS A "TOOL" IN DEVELOPING HEALTH CONCEPTS

The previous discussions give some indication of the extent to which mathematics concepts are inherent in those of health. The development of these health concepts and others involving quantitative thinking are dependent to a large extent upon the children's ability to apply appropriate mathematics concepts and to use the necessary basic number skills. A relatively large number of mathematics activities for K-3 and 4-6 grade levels are included in the following pages. It should be understood that the activities presented here by no means exhaust the possibilities. Teachers should use their own resourcefulness and ingenuity when planning mathematics activities to develop and extend concepts.

CONCEPTS	ACTIVITIES

Grades K-3

Foods and Nutrition

CONCEPTS	ACTIVITIES
Measurements-value (money); counting-rational.	Count the change needed for milk or the entire school lunch.
Measurements-value (money); multiplication.	Compute the cost of milk per child for a week, a month, 180 school days.
Counting-rational.	Count the number of times one chews a bite of bread before swallowing.
Division-measurements (value of money).	Compute the cost per child for a class trip by bus to a bakery or dairy.
Measurements-time (seconds, minutes).	Have each child keep a record of the time it takes to eat a full lunch from the cafeteria. Find the average amount of time.
Measurements-volume (pint, quart, gallon).	Compare the volume of the different types of containers in which milk is sold.
Counting-rational-quantity.	List a number of different kinds of fresh fruit available in a food store.
Measurement-time (hours).	Have children record on a clock the time of each meal; figure the lapse of time between meals.

Exercise and Physical Activity

CONCEPTS	ACTIVITIES
Counting-rote and rational.	Jump rope and count the number of jumps that can be made without missing.
Addition-carrying.	Give each child three chances to jump; add to find the total number of jumps.
Subtraction-borrowing.	Subtract the smaller number of times a child hops on one foot from the number of times he or she hopped on the other.
Addition-carrying.	Give each child three turns at bouncing a ball; add to find the total number of times the ball was bounced.

Anne	Bill
12	15
19	16
14	17
45	48

CONCEPTS	ACTIVITIES
Counting-rational; multiplication.	Count the number of breaths taken in one minute; find the number of breaths taken in an hour.

Sleep, Rest, Relaxation

Counting-rational; addition and division	While relaxing count the number of heartbeats in one minute; in two minutes, in three minutes; add; find the average per minute.

Safety

Counting-rote and rational	Count the number of street crossings on the way to school.
Counting-addition with carrying.	Count the number of street crossing on the way to school that have safety patrols, policemen, or crossing guards.
The number system.	Have each child copy his or her telephone number and bring it to school; make a class telephone directory; add the telephone number of the school and fire department to the directory; learn how to read and write telephone numbers.

The Human Organism, Its Structure, Function and Care

Measurements-weight (lb.); subtraction; vocabulary development-1b., pounds.	Teach the children how to weigh themselves; have them keep an individual record of their weight by months. Subtract to find the gain in weight from month to month, and gain for the nine school months; learn the abbreviation for pounds.
Measurement-linear (ft. in.); subtraction with number line; vocabulary development feet (ft.) inch (in.)	Teach the children to read a measuring tape; have them keep an individual record of their height by months; use a number line to find the increase in height during the nine school months; learn the abbreviations for feet and inches.
Measurement-temperature.	Check the classroom thermometer at regular intervals during the day in order to maintain healthful classroom temperature.
Counting-rational	Count the number of various parts of the body, such as joints, fingers, teeth, arms, legs, toes, and so on.
Quantity.	List by number the ways germs get from one person to another.
Comparisons.	Record and compare the number of times per day one cares for the body by brushing teeth, washing hands, combing hair, cleaning fingernails, and so on.

Grade Levels 4-6
Foods and Nutrition

Comparison of prices.	Study the price lists of foods to determine the best buys.
Fractions.	Compute the cost of 1 1/2 lb. grapes, 2 3/4 lb. oranges, and the like, needed for making a fresh fruit salad for the class.
Relationships.	Compute the savings on foods purchased in large cans as compared with small cans.
Measurements-weight, liquid, numbers.	List fruits and vegetables sold by the pound; note other measures used to sell fruits and vegetables, such as pint, quart, peck, bushel, and dozen; compare the amount of lima beans in a pint with the amount that weighs one pound.
Measurements-liquids.	Find the number of gallons of milk one drinks in a month by drinking a quart a day; compute as denominate numbers.
Measurements-dry, liquid; fractions; multiplication.	Measure the ingredients needed to make bread; find the fractional and multiple parts of the recipe.
Addition; subtraction.	List the most common foods and the total calories for each; with the children, arrive at the approximate number of calories each child needs for the day; have the children keep a daily record of their caloric intake from food at each meal and between snacks.

Exercise and Physical Activity

Measurements-area of square feet (sq. ft.)	Mark off a softball diamond; find the area of the diamond; arrive at the formula a =1xw (area equals length times width).
Measurements-linear.	Measure the chest expansion before and after a deep breath.
Comparison.	Compare the number of heartbeats and pulse rate before and after vigorous exercise.
Measurements-linear.	Use a pedometer to learn the distance covered during a physical education period.

Sleep, Rest, Relaxation

Addition; division, comparison.	Find the average heartbeat per minute when relaxing; compare with number of heartbeats after vigorous exercise.
Fractions.	Compute the fraction of a total day spent in sleep, rest, and relaxation.
Percentage.	Compute the percentage of a day set aside for sleeping.

Safety

Graphs-circle; fractions.	Construct a circle graph to show fraction of children who walk, ride buses, or ride bicycles to school.
Graphs-line; fractions.	Make a line graph to show distances children live from school; the number and place of entrances and exits to the building.
Graphs-bar.	Have children prepare a graph to show where school accidents occurred last year; these areas might include on the playground, inside the school building, en route to and from school, and so on.

The Human Organism, its Structure, Function and Care

Measurements-area (sq. ft.); division.	Find the area of the classroom and determine the amount of floor space available per child.
Measurements-volume (cu. ft.)	Find the number of cubic feet in the classroom and determine amount of air space; inductively arrive at the formula v=lxwxh (volume equals length times width times height); find the average amount of air space per child.
Graphs-line; percentage; average.	Have each child make a line graph to show his or her weight in feet and inches as recorded on the first Monday of each month; figure the percentage of weight increase from October to May; find the average amount of weight gained each month.
Measurements-linear; percentage.	Have each child make a line graph to show his or her height in feet and inches as recorded on the first Monday of each month; figure the percentage of increase between October and May.

Graphs-line.	Make a line graph to show height in feet and inches of the entire class when standing with backs against the wall; find the median height..
Graphs-line	Make a line graph to show the height in feet and inches of the entire class when seated with backs against the wall; find the median height.
Graphs-line.	Make a line graph to show the length in feet and inches from wall to end of each child's heel when the class is seated with backs against the wall; find the median length.
Measurements-linear; comparison; reading and interpreting graphs.	Compare the line graphs of the children when standing and seated to note the tallest child, the shortest child, and the child with the longest legs, and so on.
Graphs-circle	Have the children make a circle graph to show the results of their recent vision tests.
Measurements-temperature.	Learn how to read a clinical thermometer to note the range of body temperature.

The preceding activities have proved useful in various field tested situations in the development of concepts.

SUGGESTIONS FOR SUPPLEMENTARY READING

Blake, S., et al, Mathematical problem solving and young children, *Early Childhood Education Journal*, 81-4, Winter 1995.

Bradsby, S. and Bradsby, L. Math program helps teachers monitor success of every child, *Thrust for Educational Leadership*, 18-19, October 1995.

Gierl, J. and Bisanz, J., Anxieties and Attitudes Related to Mathematics in Grades 3 and 6, *The Journal of Experimental Education*, 139-158, Winter 1995.

James, D.C.S., and Adams, T.L., Connecting nutrition and mathematics: the 5-a-day for better health plan, *Journal of School Health*, 119, March 1996.

Kamii, C., et al., Fourth graders invent ways of computing averages, *Teaching Children Mathematics*, 78-83, October 1996.

Kostecky, J. and Roe, L., Generating excitement with math projects, *Teaching Pre K-8*, 62-3, January 1996.

Lewis, C. and Lewis, T., Getting acquainted, *Teaching Children Mathematics*, 24-5, September 1996.

Mitchell, C.E., et al., Scientific methodology and elementary school mathematics, *School Science and Mathematics*, 260-3, May 1995.

Ross, K., Grocery-store math, *Learning 94*, 94, September 1994.

Thomas, D, Math games, *Childhood Education*, 15, November/December 1995.

CHAPTER 8

INTEGRATION OF HEALTH AND SCIENCE

The health program and the science program in the elementary schools are characterized by divergent yet somewhat similar practices. These practices are evident from the available textbooks, recent curriculum guides, and teaching units used in some classrooms. For instance, some publishers offer separate series of health and science textbooks. Other publishers have science-health series for the elementary schools. Further examination reveals separate curriculum guides in health and science as a part of the total social studies program. Teaching units follow the same practices; that is, there are separate units for health and for science, or ones integrating health and science. One generalization seems rather apparent; that is, there is a common agreement that health and science are essential, and that both should be included in the curriculum offerings for elementary school children. It is the purpose of this chapter to examine the teaching of health and science, with special attention given to integration.

A fundamental tenet of science education emphasizes the relatedness of science to the total curriculum, especially in the areas of health and social studies. Through the integration of health and science, both areas can be reinforced, and the subject matter can be more functional and coherent for children. The practical application of this integration is found in current practices used by some teachers to extend and broaden concepts. Three illustrations are cited as examples. First, when children study about light (physical science) it seems appropriate to include a study of the eye (biological science or health). Second, when the human ear is being studied, learnings can be enhanced through the study of sound. Third, the study of electricity has a practical application when integrated with safety.

SCIENTIFIC METHOD OF DEVELOPING HEALTH CONCEPTS

It is common knowledge that the elementary school child possesses an intrinsic urge to learn about himself or herself and the environment. This seemingly innate desire provides self-motivation – a desirable prerequisite to effective learning. For the most part when a child wants to know, or is self-motivated, more and more questions are asked. Even before children start school they begin to ask questions. "Why Daddy?" is only the beginning of what should be a lifetime of intelligent inquiry. "Why do I get hungry when I play?" "Where does the sun go when it sets?" "Why do we grow two sets of teeth?" "Where does a light go when it goes out?" "How can medicine when swallowed stop a headache?" "Do people have to die?" "What makes it rain?" "Why do I get out of breath when I run?" Such questions are indicative of the normal, ceaseless flow of inquiry that is characteristic of the curiosity aroused and stimulated by health and science in the daily life of the elementary school child. Certainly one criterion for daily evaluation might be *how many intelligent questions* have been asked by children as a result of teaching. Through the integration of health and science, the teacher can plan meaningful experiences around the solving of problems that are significant to the children, rather than answering unimportant questions that stress the recall of unrelated scientific facts.

Health and science are *child-centered* because the subject matter comes from the everyday world of children. Also, the method of acquiring the subject matter is familiar. During the preschool years, the child uses some of the same methods used in school to find out about himself or herself and the world. After entering school the child acquires additional ways to learn. Hence, when a child is faced with a problem to solve, it is natural to ask questions, investigate, observe, manipulate, construct, experiment, read, and discuss in order to arrive at acceptable solutions and meaningful generalizations. As children grow and mature they become more skillful in these methods and function at increasingly higher levels of operation. Thus, health and science involve more than subject matter facts, and concepts; they involve a way of problem solving, a way of thinking known as the scientific method.

Health teaching might well be characterized by the use of the scientific method in the development of health concepts. Among other things this method involves two significant factors, namely, a problem and the process of solving it. In order to use the scientific method to develop health concepts, children become involved in the learning process of formulating and stating a problem. A problem is a task that a child can understand but for which he or she does not have an immediate solution.

The children are further involved in the learning process as they participate in the necessary steps of the scientific method in solving problems relating to health and science. The following three outcomes are apparent: (1) health concepts tend to be learned more thoroughly, (2) skills of scientific thinking involved in approaching and solving problems tend to become more functional, and (3) the scientific approach tends to help children develop a scientific attitude. Therefore it seems imperative that a teacher's plan include both the concept and the procedure, since the children will be learning both.

As an example, a lesson plan for Grade 6 might include the following: (1) science and health concepts previously developed with the children: food is prepared for the use in the body by the process of digestion; (2) health concept for this lesson: digestion changes food so that it can pass into the blood and be used by the cells. Guides for the teacher are followed by purposeful activities involving steps in scientific thinking.

I. Help the children to identify, define, and limit the problem.

Question decided upon with the children; how does food that we eat get into the blood?

II. Encourage children to formulate tentative hypotheses as they tell from their own experiences what they know about the problem, and what they think is the solution.

III. Guide children to suggest appropriate methods for solving the problem, and authoritative sources to use for checking accuracy and authenticity of information gathered.

Ways to Find the Answers to Today's Question:

1. Conduct an experiment.

2. Ask the school nurse to come to our classroom and talk with us on the question.

3. Locate and read in the health books about the digestive and circulatory systems.

4. Study charts showing these two systems.

5. See if we can find additional information at home.

IV. Assist children in making careful, accurate observations while gathering pertinent information.

Conduct the following experiment:

1. Remove a small piece of shell from the large end of an egg.

2. Make a small hole through both the shell and the lining in the small end of the egg.

3. Insert a small glass tube through the hole in the small end. Seal around the hole with sealing wax.

4. Place the egg in the top of a bottle with enough water to cover the larger end.

5. Observe the results the next day. (Through the process of osmosis, the liquid in the bottle passes through the membrane of the egg. The pressure of additional liquid in the egg causes displacement of some liquid in the egg tube.

V. Assist the children to appraise and verify the information.

Ask the school nurse to use charts on the digestive and circulatory systems in verifying for the children what has happened. Check the conclusions by reading several textbooks.

VI. Assist the children to summarize and organize the relevant information and to draw conclusions. Record the experiment as follows:

Purpose: How does the food that we eat get into the blood?

Materials: Egg, small glass tube, sealing wax, bottle, water.

Procedures:

1. Remove a small piece of shell from the large end of an egg.

2. Make a small hole through both the shell and the lining in the small end of the egg.

3. Insert a small glass tube through the hole in the small end. Seal around the hole with sealing wax.

4. Place the egg in the top of the bottle with enough water to cover the larger end.

5. Observe the results the next day.

Observations:

The water passed through the lining of the egg.

Conclusions:

Based on the observations of the experiment, the statements made by the school nurse, and the information from health and science books, the following conclusions seem warranted. The digested food passes through the wall of the blood vessels of the stomach and intestines in much the same way that the water passed through the lining of the egg.

VII. Plan ways with the children to use the information in solving other problems.

1. Make a list of foods that are easily digested.

2. Discuss why infants are given liquid or soft diets.

3. Plan a day's menu for a convalescent person.

Obviously, one of the basic aims of elementary education should be to teach children how to think. According to this premise, the children need to study the reasoning process, or the way they arrived at the solution to their problem. For instance, under the teacher's direction, the children might prepare a guide to follow in certain learning situations that center around problem solving. The following is submitted as an example of this procedure.

STEPS WE USE TO SOLVE PROBLEMS

1. We discuss our problem and state it in question form.

2. We discuss what we know about the problem. We attempt to make sensible guesses about the solution.

3. We list how and where we get the information on the particular problem.

4. We gather information.

5. We check the information to be sure that it is accurate and authentic.

6. We record the answers we accept.

7. We use the information.

This discussion should not be interpreted to mean that every time a health or science problem arises these steps should be followed verbatim or that, when used, every step should be taken for the problem approached. However, if children have intelligent guidance, they can make great progress in the ability to solve problems in this manner.

For the most part, through the study of health and science, children can experience the scientific way of thinking. In other words, while developing health concepts the children practice skills needed in everyday life situations involving (1) making wise choices, (2) drawing valid conclusions, and (3) making intelligent decisions. Thus, it is hoped that behavior is influenced to the extent that the children begin to develop scientific attitudes. Among the desirable behavioral changes would be a tendency on the part of the child to:

1. Not jump to conclusions
2. Look for reliable sources for information
3. Respect authorities
4. Maintain an inquiring and open mind
5. Evaluate a mistake as a step toward achievement
6. Change his or her mind when discovering he or she is wrong
7. Face problems rather than avoid them
8. Think before acting rather than act and thinking later
9. Feel optimistic about his or her own ability to solve problems

ACTIVITIES INVOLVING THE INTEGRATION OF HEALTH AND SCIENCE

Children learn about health and science in many ways. Experimentation and/or demonstration are successful ways for helping children develop health concepts. In addition, experiments and demonstrations can lead to other ways of learning. After completing an experiment, and observing and noting the results, children need to turn to authoritative sources to check their conclusions. Therefore, they read, use visual aids (including the Internet, if available), hold interviews, take field trips, and the like, in order to appraise and verify the information before drawing conclusions.

The opportunities for integrating health and science are numerous. The resourceful teacher is limited only by imagination and ingenuity. As an example, in the following simulated fourth-grade lesson a science demonstration is used to introduce a unit on disease.

Teacher: What do you suppose would happen if I took a plant and put a cover over it for a day or two?

Child: It would die.

Teacher: Why?

Child: No air.

Teacher: (Writes the word *air* on the board.) Yes, it needs air in order to live.

Teacher: We also need air in order to live. Now, let us take a deep breath and hold it. (Pause) See, you cannot hold it very long because you need air to breathe. We know that living things need air, but where do we find air?

Child: Everywhere.

Teacher: Yes, just about everywhere.

Teacher: Can you see air?

Child: No.

Teacher: Can you hear air?

Child: Yes, sometimes.

Teacher: Let's see if we can show that air is in many places. Why do you suppose I can't push this egg in this bottle? (Teachers uses a bottle with a slightly smaller opening than the hard boiled egg.)

Child: Air keeps it out.

Teacher: Now I want you to look closely and listen. (Teacher puts a piece of burning paper in the bottle. One end of the egg is placed in the mouth of the bottle. If the experiment is successful the egg is "sucked" into the bottle.)

Teacher: Now what do you think happened?

(Children form hypothesis.)

Teacher; Three things happened: First, some of the warm air is expanded in the bottle and pushed out around the egg; second, when the rest of the air cooled inside the bottle, that air contracted; third, the air outside in trying to get in pushed the egg into the bottle. Can you suggest how we might get the egg out?

Child: Try to blow into the bottle (Teacher tips bottle up, blows hard into it, and removes mouth quickly. If the experiment is successful, the egg should be forced out of the bottle by air.)

Teacher: Why do you think the egg came out of the bottle?

Child: The pressure of the air blown into the bottle pushed the egg out.

Teacher: So we see that air is not only just about everywhere, but that it also has pressure, and has great force to get into places.

Teacher: Let's read something else interesting about air. Open you health textbook to the table of contents and find the chapter dealing with disease. Read the selection silently to find out about some tiny enemies of the body. (Children read silently. Teacher assists children with new and difficult words.)

Teacher: Did you find out?

Child: Yes.

Teacher: What are these tiny enemies called?

Child: Germs.

Teacher: (Writes the word *germs* on the board.) Where are they found?

Child: In the air, in water, in the soil, and in the body.

Teacher: Today, we learned many places where air is found, and that we need air in order to live. We read in our books that tiny enemies called germs are in the air, as well as other places. Now what sort of problems does that present for us? Let's try in the next few days to learn many things about germs. To begin let us see what some of the class members would like to find out about germs. (Children write their own questions on the board.) How would you like to work on these problems? How should we go about solving this problem? This problem? (And so on.)

SCIENCE CONCEPTS INHERENT IN TEACHING ABOUT HEALTH

Thus far it has been suggested that (1) health and science subject matter can be integrated, and (2) the development of the scientific way of thinking can be inherent in the methods the teacher uses with the children to develop the concepts. With this in mind, certain specific science concepts that are inherent in both health and science have been selected as examples of integration.

FOODS AND NUTRITION

Concept: Air is essential to life.

Experiment: Air can enter a plant through the leaf.

Procure a leaf with a long stalk attached and seal it into a hole through a cork. Fit this with a side tube, and seal the cork into a flask containing water. Suck air from the side of the tube. Air bubbles will be seen to issue from the end of the stalk.

Experiment: To show the respiration of a plant. Place the plant in a test tube held in a weighted wooden block. Put this in a bowl containing lime water and cover the plant with a jar. Keep the plant in a dark place for several hours or examine it the next day. The lime water will be milky, showing that carbon dioxide was given off; the rise in the level shows that a considerable amount of oxygen was taken in.

Activity: Discuss the reasons for the pressurized cabins on airplanes and submarines. Discuss problems of air pressure for space travel.

Concept: Living things produce their kind in a variety of ways.

Experiment: Observing the development of flowers into fruit. Collect specimens of flowers in different stages of maturity, from newly opened buds to specimens in which the petals have fallen. Cut each ovary open and note the changes that occur during the seed development.

Look over a quart of freshly picked peas or string beans and pick out the pods that are not completely filled. Open these and compare them with fully filled specimens. The abortive seeds are the remains of the ovules that were not fertilized by pollen.

Concept: Chemical changes play an important part in our lives.

Experiment: Testing food for starch. Cut open a potato. Apply diluted iodine to its surface Mix a small amount of cornstarch in water. Apply the diluted iodine to the mixture; also apply it to a slice of bread and a small amount of milk. Cut open an orange. Apply the iodine to its surface. (The change of color to bluish purple indicates the presence of starch.)

Experiment: Testing food for carbohydrates. Cut open an apple. Apply Benedict's solution to its surface; also apply the solution to a soda cracker. Heat some raisins in water, then apply the solution. (The change of color to blue indicates the presence of sugar.)

Experiment: Testing for protein.

Apply copper sulfate and washing soda to a slice of bread; apply copper sulfate and washing soda to a small amount of peanut butter; apply copper sulfate and washing soda to a slice of cheese. (The change of color to red indicates the presence of protein.)

Experiment: Testing for acids.

1. Test a small amount of vinegar with blue litmus paper.

2. Test a small amount of grapefruit juice with blue litmus paper.

3. Test a small amount of lemon juice with blue litmus paper.

4. Test a small amount of sour milk with blue litmus paper. (The change of color of the blue litmus paper to red indicates the presence of acid.)

Activity: Make a chart to record the facts learned about the foods tested. Mark an X to show the materials each food contains.

Materials in Foods

Foods	*Acids*	*Protein*	*Starch*	*Sugar*
Bread			X	
Crackers				X
Milk				
Cheese				
Potatoes				
Apples				
Grapefruit				
Oranges				
Raisins				
Peanut Butter				

SLEEP, REST AND RELAXATION

Concept: The body needs rest and oxygen.

Experiment: To show the effect of exercise on the pulse. Have each child select a partner. Have them take each other's pulse rate at rest and after vigorous exercise.

Activity: Record the results and draw conclusions.

SAFETY

Concept: Fire out of control is a very destructive force.

Experiment: How a fire extinguisher works. To demonstrate the action of a fire extinguisher use baking soda and vinegar. Place a tablespoon of baking soda in a drinking glass and slowly pour vinegar on it. The bubbles will be extinguished. This should be a teacher-demonstrated experiment, because it involves the use of matches.

Concept: Electrical energy can be converted into other forms of energy-heat, light, motion, and sound.

Experiment: How a flashlight works. Wrap the end of a short piece of bell wire around the base of the bulb. Set the bulb firmly on the center terminal of a flashlight cell. Press the free end of the wire against the bottom of the cell.

Activities: Show how a fuse works and why it is necessary. Discuss the benefits and hazards resulting from modern household electrical appliances. Demonstrate the safe use of household electrical appliances.

CLOTHING

Concept: Changes in air conditions determine the weather.

Experiment: To show how a thermometer registers temperature of air.

Part 1. Place an electric fan near a dish of ice cubes. Place a thermometer in a position to receive the air being blown over the ice cubes. Note the temperature. Relate this information to the kinds of clothes to wear on cold days.

Part 2. Place a thermometer near the hot air coming from a boiling tea kettle. Note the temperature. Relate this information to the kinds of clothes to wear.

Note: As a safety precaution when an electric fan or boiling water is used, it may be advisable that the teacher conduct the experiment while the children make the observations.

Activity: Discuss the reasons why an electric fan can make one feel cooler during summer heat.

Experiment: To show how a thermometer works. Fill a thin glass bottle with colored water. Insert a long glass tube through the small hole in the cork stopper. Place the hands around the bottle. The heat of the hands should warm the water and cause it to rise in the tube.

THE HUMAN ORGANISM - ITS STRUCTURE, FUNCTION AND CARE

Concept: The body is a wonderful mechanism that performs many duties.

Experiment: To test the sense of smell. Have children seated at their desks facing the front of the room. Have windows and doors of the room closed for the few minutes it takes to perform this experiment. From the back of the room, pour about two tablespoonfuls of household ammonia on a piece of cheesecloth. Ask the children to raise their hands as soon as an odor is detected.

Activity: Discuss ways the sense of smell can protect us from danger. Compare the various mechanisms of the body to a machine. Demonstrate how the joints give leverage to the body. Demonstrate how muscles give flexibility to the body.

Concept: The organs of the body work together as a unit.

Experiment: Have the school nurse visit the class and demonstrate the use of a stethoscope. The children can use it to listen to the heart action.

Activity: This experiment should lead naturally into a discussion of what the heart does and its importance in maintaining good health. Activities that might injure the heart and diseases that sometimes result in heart impairment might also be discussed.

Experiment: To observe the pulse beat. Place a thumbtack in the large end of a toothpick. Hold the hand out with the palm up and the wrist level. Place the head of the thumbtack on the wrist at the point where the pulse is felt. Observe the toothpick as it moves each time that the heart beats.

Concept: Light is bent or refracted when it passes from a medium of one density to another.

Experiment: A water-drop microscope. Place a drop of water carefully on a plate of glass. Bring your eye close to the drop and look at something small through the water drop and glass. This serves as a simple microscope.

Experiment: Making a coin appear with refraction. Place a coin in the bottom of a teacup on a table. Stand away and arrange your line of vision so that the edge of the cup just interferes with your seeing the coin in the bottom. Hold this position while another person pours water carefully into the cup.

Activity: What do you observe: How do you account for this? Apply this information to a study of the camera. Discuss lenses of eyeglasses used for farsightedness, nearsightedness, and astigmatism.

Concept: Pitch depends upon the number of vibrations per sound made by the sounding body.

Experiment: To note the vibration of objects.

Part 1. Run a toy fire truck with a siren turned on. The faster the truck runs, the higher the note it produces.

Part 2. Blow across the mouth of empty bottles of different shapes and sizes to note the sounds produced.

Concept: The respiratory system supplies oxygen to the body and gets rid of carbon dioxide.

Experiment: To show that expired air contains carbon dioxide. Put some clear lime water in a glass jar. Place the end of a glass tube in the lime water and blow through it for a few minutes. The lime water turns milky when it comes in contact with carbon dioxide.

The above examples provide just a few of the almost unlimited possibilities of integrating health and science. Teachers can use their own resourcefulness and ingenuity to expand these examples manyfold.

SUGGESTIONS FOR SUPPLEMENTARY READING

Barrow, L.H., et al., Evening science: solving science problems, *Science and Children*, 34, October 1996, p. 20-3.

Germann, P.J. and Aram, R.J., Student performance on the science processes of recording data, analyzing data, drawing conclusions, and providing evidence, *Journal of Research in Science Teaching*, 33, September 1996, p. 773-98.

Huber, R.A. and Walker, B.L., Science reading do's and dont's, *Science Scope*, 20, October 1996, p. 22-3.

Jarman, R. and McAleese, L., A survey of children's reported use of school science in their everyday lives, *Research in Education*, 55, May 1996, p. 1-15.

Kamen, M., A teacher's implementation of authentic assessment in an elementary science classroom, *Journal of Research in Science Teaching*, 33, October 1996, p. 859-77.

Kolstad, R.K., et al., Better teaching of science through integration, *Journal of Instructional Psychology*, 22, June 1995, p. 130-4.

Metz, K.E., Reassessment of developmental constraints on children's science instruction, *Review of Educational Research*, 65, Summer 1995, p. 93-127.

Royce, C.A. and Wiley, D.A., Children's literature and the teaching of science: possibilities and cautions, *Clearing House*, 70, September/October 1996, p. 18-20.

Van Sickle, M.L., and Dickman, C.B., Science across the disciplines, *Science Scope*, 20, November/December 1996, p. 22-4.

Wise, K.C., Strategies for teaching science: what works? *Clearing House*, 69, July/August 1996, p. 337-8.

CHAPTER 9

INTEGRATION OF HEALTH AND SOCIAL STUDIES

Throughout life, human beings are involved in the processes of social relationships. In our democratic society, human relationships, rights, and responsibilities constitute basic human values set forth as basic tenets. Thus, it follows that the philosophy of education includes expressions of the belief that each individual be afforded opportunities for optimum growth socially, as well as intellectually, physically, and emotionally. To this end, the school as an agency in a democracy is charged with the responsibility of offering experiences through which the individual grows and develops in his or her ability to function effectively as a participating member of society.

Social education is a broad term that refers in general to all of the experiences that contribute to the child's social learning. However, for purposes of this discussion, social education in the elementary school will be limited to the social learning situations inherent in the subjects of health and social studies.

In general, educators consider social studies to include all of our group skills and attitudes, all the knowledge of our interdependence with others and with nature, all of our social customs and mores, and all of our moral and spiritual values as they affect our living with others.

There is some difference of opinion concerning the number of different subjects to be taught in the block of time that is assigned daily to the teaching of social studies. On the other hand, there seems to be rather common agreement among educators that geography, history, and civics constitute the major subjects in the social studies program for the elementary school. Among other things, this postulation is predicated upon certain generalizations, as follows:

1. From a study of the subject matter taught in the areas of geography, history, and civics, it is hoped that children will arrive at basic concepts needed in becoming *well-informed members* of a democratic society.
2. Through the teaching of social sciences involving individuals interacting with others in their environment, it is hoped that children will gain competencies in the *processes of socialization.*
3. Through the use of appropriate methods in the teaching of social sciences it is hoped that children will have opportunities to grow and develop in their abilities to use procedures needed to function effectively as *participating members* in a democratic society.

In this context, health and social studies have a high degree of compatibility in at least two important respects. That is, both are concerned with (1) the kind of environment in which learning takes place, and (2) the quality of the learning experiences. Succinctly stated, the integration of health and social studies involves relating children to the environment in which they find themselves to the end that they and their environment may profit from the interaction.

SOCIAL HEALTH CLIMATE IN THE CLASSROOM

The role of the child in the classroom might well serve as an identifying characteristic of any system of education. Based on the values placed upon the dignity and worth of the individual, the classroom in the modern elementary school should serve as a laboratory for human relations and be representative of a miniature democratic society. Learning thus becomes a matter of personal meaning to the individual.

In the past, intelligence to some extent has been thought of as a somewhat static quality, remaining throughout life within a rather narrowly measured range. However, if the quality and frequency of experiences through time tend to increase the individual's personal discovery of meaning, one might expect the individual to operate at increasingly higher intellectual levels. With the increased importance that perceptual psychology attaches to the significance of increasing the depth, richness, and extent of experience, the classroom teacher faces the task of improving the quality of the educational experiences offered children in the classroom.

UNIT TEACHING IN HEALTH AND SOCIAL STUDIES

Thus far it has been pointed out that the social health climate of the classroom used in the teaching of health and social studies contributes to the total growth and development of children in a democratic society. With this thought in mind, it is more readily understood why the unit method is an effective procedure for teaching health and social studies. Among its many advantages, unit teaching lends itself to:

1. Democratic practices and procedures in the classroom
2. Individualization of instruction
3. Many kinds of achievement at many levels
4. Development of the uniqueness of the individual
5. Identification and development of talents and special abilities among children
6. Development of feelings of security, adequacy and belongingness among the children
7. Learning experiences appropriate to each stage of child development with its accompanying developmental tasks
8. Integration of the physical, social, intellectual, and emotional aspects of the individual.

HEALTH CONCEPTS INHERENT IN SOCIAL STUDIES CONTENT

The teaching of health and social studies deals with the child in his or her educative process. The discussion thus far espouses the democratic processes employed in the teaching of health and social studies. In addition to the procedures used for teaching there is yet another relevant facet of integration. An analysis of the concepts in the social studies curriculum indicates the importance placed upon the teaching of health by including health content as an integral part of the social studies curriculum. Such integration enhances the effectiveness of social learnings for the child by strengthening, extending, and giving depth, meaning, and pertinence to the knowledge needed as an intelligent, informed person. Since health involves the functioning of human beings in their total environment, it seems logical to assume that not only the knowledge and wisdom derived from a study of geography, history, and civics, but from mathematics, science, art, music, and physical education needs to be integrated with health.

With the present knowledge of child growth and development, and how learning is internalized, the *approach* to what children learn takes on new and added significance if the objectives of social studies are to be realized.

In general, educators tend to agree on the following objectives of social studies:

1. Development of skills and abilities to be used in cooperative group participation.
2. Development of concepts important to carrying out responsibilities at increasing levels of maturity.
3. Development of skills and abilities that are important to good human relations.
4. Development of critical-thinking and problem-solving skills and abilities.

An analysis of these objectives indicates the emphasis of the social studies program in the elementary school to be upon the life experience of the child. In this context, certain aspects of health become an integral part of the social studies program.

Social studies involve more than the teaching of separate subjects such as geography, history, civics, and the like. The discipline involves integration of various subjects, each contributing to the objectives as stated. To illustrate this point, parts of a resource unit on clothing are given. This particular topic was selected because (1) clothing is rather generally accepted as a social studies topic, with subject matter appearing in the most widely used social studies textbook series for the elementary school, (2) clothing represents a need of people everywhere, and (3) clothing is also a health topic.

RESOURCE UNIT-CLOTHING (GRADE 3)

Subject Matter Area	Concepts	Content
Health	Clothing is one of man's basic needs.	A. Why do we wear clothing?
Health	Clothes protect the body.	1. How does clothing meet bodily needs?
Health	Clothes satisfy certain social needs.	2. How does clothing satisfy social needs?
Social Studies	The sources of clothing are numerous and varied.	B. What are the sources of our clothing?
Social studies	The knowledge and skills of many people are necessary for the production of materials for clothing.	
Mathematics	Much time is required to produce the materials for clothing.	

PART I-ANIMALS

ANIMALS THAT GIVE US WOOL

Geography-Science	Climatic conditions are a determining factor in the producing of wool.	1. Which animals give us wool? 2. Where are the wool producing areas?
Science	The raising of sheep for	3. How are sheep

	wool requires special knowledge and skills. clothing?	raised to produce wool for
Science	The fleece is spun into yarn which is used to make woolen cloth.	4. How is raw wool made ready for the mills?
		5. What happens to the fleece at the mills?
History	Methods of making woolen cloth improve from time to time.	6. How is woolen yarn made into cloth?
Health	We wear many articles of clothing made from wool.	7. What articles of clothing are made of wool?

ANIMALS THAT GIVE US LEATHER

Science	Birds, fishes, mammals, and reptiles produce leather for clothing.	1. What animals give us leather for clothing?
Science	Numerous processes are used in making leather.	2. What processes are used for making leather?
Social studies	Articles of clothing made from leather serve many purposes.	3. What articles of clothing are made of leather?

PART II – PLANT

COTTON

Science	Cotton is a plant.	1. How is cotton raised?
Geography, Science	Cotton grows in a warm climate.	2. Where is cotton raised?
Geography, Science	Much of the south has a mild climate, abundant rainfall, and a long growing season.	
Geography	Cotton is among the most important crops raised in the south.	
Science, History	The invention of the cotton gin greatly increased cotton-raising in the south.	3. How is cotton prepared for the mill?
Science, History	Modern machines made cotton into cloth.	4. How is cotton made into cloth?
Science, History, Mathematics	Articles of cotton are not as expensive today as in the past, because new machines have greatly lowered its cost.	5. What articles of clothing are made of cotton?

RUBBER

Science	Rubber is a plant.	1. How is rubber raised?
Geography	Rubber comes from trees that grow in warm, rainy climates.	2. Where is rubber raised?
Science	Numerous processes are involved from the time rubber sap leaves the tree	3. How is rubber made into articles of

	until it is made into an article of clothing.	clothing?
Science	Some clothing accessories are made of pure rubber. Synthetic rubber is used also.	4. What articles of clothing are made of rubber?

PART III – SYNTHETICS

Science	Rayon, nylon, dacron, and other synthetics are used for making clothing.	1. What synthetics are used for making clothing?
Science, Geography	Many materials used today are made from wood pulp, milk, soybeans, and coal.	2. Of what are synthetics made?
Science	Synthetics are man-made by "putting together" materials.	3. What does the word *synthetic* mean?
Science	Many articles of clothing are made from synthetics.	4. What articles of clothing are made of synthetics?
Science, Social Studies	Synthetics have special characteristics that make them attractive to the buyer.	5. Why are synthetics an increasing source of clothing?
Science	Synthetics are becoming increasingly important as a source of our clothing.	
Science, Social Studies	Cloth from clothing goes from the mills to the factories. Many processes are used in the making of clothes.	C. How are clothes made? 1. Where are clothes made? 2. What processes are

		used in making clothes?
Social Studies	Clothing can be made in clothing factories, at a tailor shop, or at home.	
Social Studies	Clothing factories supply clothing to the wholesale house.	D. How are clothes bought and sold?
Social Studies	Wholesale houses buy and sell in large quantities.	1. How do articles of clothing get from factories to retail stores?
Social Studies	Retail stores buy clothing to sell from the wholesale houses.	
Social Studies	We are dependent upon the employees of distributing houses and stores to make clothing available to us.	2. What services are provided by retail stores in selling clothes to us?
Social Studies	Displays, advertisements and sales persons help people know which clothing is for sale.	
Health, Science,	People select clothing on the basis of style, color, wearing qualities, cost, and the season of the year or the place where the clothing is to be worn.	3. What factors are considered in purchasing clothes?
Mathematics	Many factors determine the price of clothing.	
Health	We have the responsibility to prevent undue wear and soiling of our clothes.	E. How are clothes cared for?

		1. How can we maintain the appearance and durability of our clothes?
Health	The care of our clothes to make them feel better, look better, and last longer is the joint responsibility of ourselves our parents, and other people.	2. How do others help us care for our clothes?
Social Studies	Boys and girls of many countries wear clothes. like ours	F. What kinds of clothes are worn by people around the world?
Geography	Latitude, nearness to bodies of water, direction of winds, and altitudes influence climate.	1. What kinds of clothes are worn in hot, wet climates?
Geography	Climate influences the clothes people wear.	2. What kinds of clothes are worn in and near the frigid zone?
Health, History	Festive occasions mean "dress up" time.	3. What kinds of clothes are worn by children in different countries for festive occasions?

SOCIAL STUDIES ACTIVITIES INVOLVING HEALTH

Through integration, certain health concepts tend to take on new and added meanings for the individual. Frequently, health resource units and teaching units include activities involving the social studies. To illustrate this integration, examples of geography, history and civic activities are listed.

FOODS AND NUTRITION

Make a pictorial map to show foods that are characteristic of particular countries throughout the world (geography).

Make a study of the food habits of people in other countries of the world to note the influence of geographical conditions on kinds of food available (geography).

Select a dinner menu and find the possible geographical location where each food might have been grown (geography).

On a political-physical map for each geographical region of the United States locate the region where Vitamin C foods are prevalent (geography).

Make a food-products map for each geographical region of the United States (geography)

Study the geographical distribution of foods (geography).

Make a table model relief map of the United States. Use appropriate symbols to indicate grain-, fruit-, dairy-, vegetable-, and wheat-producing areas (geography).

Study the geographical conditions necessary to raise sugar cane and sugar beets (geography).

Compare a breakfast menu of the 1790s with a breakfast of today (history).

Trace the origin of some of the foods we eat today, such as corn bread and succotash (history).

EXERCISE AND PHYSICAL ACTIVITY

Learn games, dances, and relays from different countries of the world. Locate
countries in which these activities originated (geography).

Learn dances and games from colonial days (history).

Trace the history of the Olympic games and discuss their value (history).

SLEEP, REST, RELAXATION

Mark time belts on a map of the world. Indicate what time it is in you locality
when children in each of the other time belts might be going to bed
(geography).

Make a study of the kinds of beds and bed coverings used in other countries
(geography).

Discuss the siesta. Relate this practice to climatic conditions (geography).

SAFETY

Make a series of safety maps including school grounds and neighborhood
(geography).

Have map legends include symbols for
    School map;
        Halls
        Stairways
        Exits from building
        Direction of traffic
        Fire alarm boxes
    School ground map:
        Hard top area
        Grass area
        Parking area
        Playground equipment
        Areas designated for different activities

Directions for flow of traffic to and from physical education and recess period

Neighborhood map:

> Roads
> Streets
> Sidewalks
> Traffic signals
> Road signs
> Marks on road
> Safety patrol or police protected intersections

Make a spot map of your neighborhood showing types and places of accidents (geography). Indicate which accidents might have been avoided if traffic regulations had been obeyed or pedestrians had not been careless (civics).

Organize a bicycle club. Write a code of behavior for bicycle riders (civics).

Practice reporting fires and participate in fire drills (civics).

Make a survey of school and home for possible fire hazards (civics).

Visit a fire station to learn ways to prevent fires and to cooperate with firemen (civics).

Write notes to policeman, firemen, and safety patrol members to express appreciation for their protection (civics).

CLOTHING

Study rainfall and temperature maps to note conditions favorable to the growing of flax (geography).

Locate zones and hemispheres on a globe. Discuss the clothing which might be worn by children in each hemisphere and zone when it is New Year's Day in your community (geography).

Using an outline map of the world, make a pictorial map to show the areas where wool and cotton are produced (geography).

Study the dress of peoples in various parts of the world to note geographical influences on clothing (geography).

Give oral reports on Eli Whitney, James Hargreaves, and other inventors who have contributed to the growth of the textile industry (history).

Compare clothes worn by children in colonial days with clothes worn by
   children today (history)

THE HUMAN ORGANISM – ITS STRUCTURE, FUNCTION, AND CARE

Trace the history of bathing, including such items as the introduction of soap,
   bathtubs, showers, (history).

HEALTH SERVICES

Play the role of nurse and doctor who are administering immunization "shots"
   to children (civics.)
Discuss the significance of pure food and drug laws and other health
   legislation (civics).
Survey the health problems existing in your community (civics).
Discuss health problems related to specific geographical areas (geography).
Study the history of the following (history):
   Use of antiseptics (Lister)
   Discovery of microscope (Leeuwenhock)
   Discovery of Xray (Roentgen)
   Discovery of vaccination (Jenner)
Discuss the evolution of hospitals and medical and nursing profession
   (history).

SUGGESTIONS FOR SUPPLEMENTARY READING

Berson, M.J., Effectiveness of computer technology in the social studies,
   Journal of Research On Computing in Education, 28, Summer 1996, p.
   486-99.
Ediger, M., Social studies: integrating school and society, *Journal of
   Instructional Psychology*, 23, June 1996, p. 121-5.
Hope, W.C., It's time to transform social studies teaching, *The Social Studies*,
   87, July/August, 1996, p. 149-51.

Houser, N.D., Negotiating dissonance and safety for the common good: social education in the elementary classroom, *Theory and Research in Social Education*, 24, Summer 1996, p. 294-312.

McKay, R., Keep the "social" in social studies, *Canadian Social Studies*, 31, fall 1996, p. 11.

Queen, J.A., The success of 4x4 block scheduling in the social studies, *The Social Studies*, 87, November/December 1996, p. 249-53.

Sheehy, J., Multimedia: enhancing social studies programs, *Media & Methods*, 33, September/October 1996, p. 54-5.

Shields, P., Bringing the world to social studies classrooms, *Canadian Social Studies*, 31, Fall 1996, p. 54-5.

Sunal, C.S., Introducing the use of communication technology into an elementary school social studies curriculum, *International Journal of Social Education*, 10, Fall/Winter 1995-96, p. 106-23.

Wellhousen, K., Be it ever so humble: a study of homes for today's diverse society, *Young Children*, 52, November 1996, p. 72-6.

CHAPTER 10

INTEGRATION OF HEALTH AND PHYSICAL EDUCATION

Curriculum content of elementary school physical education programs usually consists of three broad categories that help to meet the recognized needs of children. These categories involve (1) active games, (2) rhythmic activities, and (3) self-testing activities. Although these categories remain much the same for all grade levels, the complexity of activities within each category increases. There is still another category that is involved in all of the above and this is the area of *basic movement and fundamental skills.* Being able to move effectively and efficiently is directly related to the proficiency with which the child will be able to perform the various fundamental motor skills. In turn, the success children will have in physical education activities will be dependent upon their proficiency of performance of these skills.

BASIC MOVEMENT AND FUNDAMENTAL SKILLS

Just as the perception of symbols is concerned with reading readiness, so is basic movement an important factor in readiness to perform in various kinds of physical education activities. Since proficient performance of physical education activities is dependent upon skill of body movement, the ability of the child to move effectively should be readily discerned. With proper teacher guidance the basic movements that the child has developed on his or her own can be improved in terms of proper principles of body mechanics and commensurate with the child's natural ability. The important factor is that in the early stages the child has been made to feel comfortable with the way he or she moves and thus is in a better position to learn correct performance of skills.

These skills involve (1) locomotor skills of walking, running, leaping, jumping, hopping, galloping, skipping, and sliding; (2) the auxiliary skills of starting, stopping, dodging, pivoting, landing, and falling; and (3) the skills of propulsion and retrieval such as throwing, striking, kicking, and catching.

ACTIVE GAMES

For purposes here games are described as *active interactions of individuals* in competitive and/or cooperative situations. This description of games places emphasis on active games as opposed to those that are passive in nature. This is to say that games in physical education are concerned with a total or near total physical response of children as they interact with each other.

In general, games played in small groups are enjoyed by most children at the K-3 level. These games ordinarily involve a few simple rules and in some cases elementary strategy. Games that involve chasing and fleeing, tag, and one small group against another, as well as those involving fundamental skills, are best suited to children at the lower elementary levels. In addition, children at this age level enjoy the game with an element of surprise, such as those that involve running for a goal on a given signal.

Children in the 4-6 level retain an interest in some of the games they played at the K-3 level, and some of them can be extended and made more difficult to meet the needs and interests of these older children. Also, games may now be introduced that call for greater bodily control, finer coordination of hands, eyes, and feet, more strength, and the utilization of some of the basic skills acquired in previous grades.

It has been found that children in the 4-6 grade level, and sometimes as low as third grade can engage satisfactorily in various types of team games such as basketball, soccer, softball, flag football, and volleyball. These games as played at the high school or college level are ordinarily too highly organized and complex for the majority of 4-6 grade level children. It is therefore necessary to modify these activities to meet the needs and interests of this age level. By way of illustration let us consider the game of basketball as played at the high school or college level. Players at these levels use the regulation size basketball of 29 1/2 inches in circumference and the goal is at a height of 10 feet. For children at the 4-6 grade level the game could be modified by using a smaller ball and lowering the goal. At this level more simple strategies also would be used in playing the game. Teachers should use their own ingenuity along with the help of children in modifying the highly organized games to adjust them for suitability for specific groups of 4-6 level children.

One approach to the introduction of the more highly organized team games is the use of preparatory games. These contain many of the same skills used in the advanced games. These games are within the capacity of children at this age level and provide them with an opportunity to learn many of the basic skills and some of the rules of the more advanced games.

RHYTHMIC ACTIVITIES

Those human movement experiences that require some sort of rhythmical accompaniment may be placed in the broad category of rhythmic activities. This description of rhythmic activities is arbitrary and is used for purposes of discussion here. Some authorities consider the meaning of the term dance to be broader than the term rhythmic activities. However, the point of view here is that there are certain human experiences that require some form of rhythmical accompaniment that do not necessarily have the same objectives as those ordinarily associated with dance. Moreover, according to my surveys, about 80 percent of the books on elementary school physical education use the term rhythmic activities while the remaining 20 percent use the term dance. It is more likely that dance is a more popular term at the secondary school and college levels.

One approach to the classification of rhythmic activities centers around the kinds of rhythmic experiences that one might wish for elementary school children to have. One such classification consists of (1) unstructured experiences, (2) semistructures experiences, and (3) structured experiences. It should be understood that in this particular way of grouping rhythmic activities a certain amount of overlapping will occur as far as the degree of structuring is concerned. Although an experience is classified as an unstructured one, there could be some small degree of structuring in some situations. With this idea in mind the following descriptions of these three types of elementary school rhythmic activities are submitted.

Unstructured experiences include those in which there is an original or creative response and in which there has been little, if any, previous explanation or discussion in the form of specific directions. The semistructured experiences include those in which certain movements or interpretations are suggested by the teacher, a child, or a group of children. Structured experiences involve the more difficult rhythmic patterns associated with the various types of dances. A well-balanced program of elementary school rhythmic activities designed to provide such experiences for children gives consideration to (1) fundamental rhythms, (2) creative rhythms, (3) movement songs (sometimes referred to as singing games, and (4) dances.

At the K-3 level fundamental rhythmic activities found in the locomotor movements of walking, running, jumping, hopping, leaping, skipping, galloping, and sliding, and the non-locomotor or axial movements such as twisting, turning, and stretching form the basis for all types of rhythmic patterns. Once the children have developed skill in the fundamental rhythms, they are ready to engage in some of the more complex dance patterns. For example, the combination of walking and hopping to musical accompaniment is the basic movement in the dance known as the schottische.

Children at the K-3 level should be given numerous opportunities to engage in creative rhythms. This kind of rhythmic activity helps them to express themselves in just the way the accompaniment "makes them feel" and gives vent to expression so necessary in the life of the child.

The movement song is a type of rhythmic activity suitable for K-3 level children. In this type of activity children can sing their own accompaniment for the various activity patterns that they use in performing the movement song.

Various kinds of dances may be included as a part of the program of rhythmic activities for the K-3 level. Ordinarily these have simple movement patterns that the child learns before progressing to some of the more complex patterns.

At the 4-6 level children can engage in rhythmic activities that are more advanced than those at the K-3 level. Creative rhythms should be continued and children should have the opportunity to create more advanced movement patterns.

Dance patterns involved in the various kinds of folk dances may be somewhat more complex, provided children have had a thorough background of fundamental rhythms and less complicated folk dances at the K-3 level. K-3 level dances can be individual activities and many of them require dancing with a partner. At the 4-6 level "couple dances" that require closer coordination of movement by partners is introduced.

SELF-TESTING ACTIVITIES

The so-called self-testing activities involve competing against one's self and natural forces. These activities are based upon the child's desire to test his or her ability in such a way that attempts are made to better performance. This is a broad term and involves such activities as stunts and tumbling, exercises with or without apparatus, and individual skill proficiency such as throwing for accuracy and/or distance, and jumping for height and distance. Some individuals have resurrected the term educational gymnastics to describe these kinds of activities. This term was used around the beginning of the 20th century and was in contrast to the term medical gymnastics, which was used to identify activities used to correct certain fundamental or organic disability or deformity. For purposes here the term self-testing activities seems more appropriate to describe this category. Moreover, in modern times about 80 percent of the elementary school physical education textbook use the term self-testing while only about 20 percent use the term educational gymnastics.

At the K-3 level, children should be given the opportunity to participate in self-testing activities that are commensurate with their ability. For example, stunts that involve imitations of animals are of great interest to boys and girls at this age level. Tumbling activities that involve some of the simple rolls are also suitable. Simple apparatus activities involving the use of such equipment as horizontal ladders, low parallel bars, low horizontal bars, and climbing ropes can be utilized.

Self-testing activities at the 4-6 level should be somewhat more advanced provided the children have had previous experience and teaching in this type of activity at the K-3 level. Tumbling activities that involve more advanced rolls and various kinds of body springs may be successfully introduced. Children at the 4-6 level may continue to take part in the apparatus activities using much the same equipment that was used at the K-3 level but moving to more advanced skills. When properly taught, apparatus activity is greatly enjoyed and is excellent for muscular development, especially for the torso and arms. Certain basic games skills are sometimes considered self-testing activities and pave the way for competence in a variety of sports. These include throwing for distance and accuracy, soccer kicking and dribbling, and throwing and catching various types of balls.

All of these broad categories of physical education activities have various degrees of effectiveness when integrated with health. The most effective, however, is in the area of active games. Therefore, the focus of this chapter will be on integration of health and active games. Before getting into some of the specific ways that health can be integrated with active games, it appears important that the reader have a clear understanding of learning through this medium.

THEORY OF ACTIVE GAME LEARNING

The active game approach to learning is concerned with how children can develop skills and concepts in the various subject areas in school while actively engaged in game situations. Although all children differ in one or more characteristics, the fact remains that they are more alike than they are different. The one common likeness of all children is that they all move; they live in a movement world, so to speak. The active game approach to learning is based essentially on the theory that children will learn better when what might be called academic learning takes place through pleasurable physical activity; that is, when the motor component operates at a maximal level in skill and concept development in school subject areas traditionally oriented to verbal learning. This is not to say that motor and verbal learning are two mutually exclusive kinds of learning, although it has been suggested that, at the two extremes, the dichotomy appears justifiable. It is recognized that in verbal learning, which involves almost complete abstract symbolic manipulations, there may be, among others, such motor components as tension, subvocal speech and physiological changes in metabolism that operate at a minimal level. It is also recognized that in active games where the learning is predominantly motor in nature, verbal learning is evident, although perhaps at a minimal level. For example, in teaching an active game there is a certain amount of verbilization in developing a kinesthetic concept of, or kinesthetic feel for, the particular game that is being taught.

The active game approach to learning is also concerned with other elements that are inherent in the participation of active games. Two such elements involve motivation, particularly as it relates to interest, and certain principles of reinforcement. These factors will be discussed in more detail in a subsequent section of the chapter, and are mentioned here only as a means of identifying the theoretical aspect of the active game approach to learning.

The procedure of learning through active games involves the selection of an active game that is taught to the children, and used as a learning activity for the development of a skill or concept in a specific subject area. An attempt is made to arrange an active learning situation so that a fundamental intellectual skill or concept is being practiced in the course of participating in the active game situation. Activities are selected that can be related to the skill or concept to be learned and which are appropriate to the physical and social abilities of the children. In order to give the reader some insight into this type of learning activity in the area of health, some representative examples follow. (Another section of the chapter will be devoted to several active games useful in the development of certain health concepts.) The first example is concerned with the concept, the skin is the first line of defense for the body against infectious agents. The game to develop the concept is Body Rebels. In the center of a large area a circle with a three-foot radius is drawn. One child is chosen to be the body, and stands in the center of the circle. Four children are selected to be the skin, and stand outside the circle. The other children are germs and station themselves about the playing area nearer the boundary lines than the skin. The germs try to run past the skin, gain entrance to the circle and tag the body. If the body is tagged, the game ends and the child who tagged the body becomes the body for the next game. If a skin tags a germ as he tries to get into the circle to reach the body, the germ must go to a line, stand still and count to ten before continuing to play. The skin tries to tag the germs only when they are near the circle. Once a germ enters the circle he is safe to tag the body.

In this game the child can dramatize that the body tries to resist bacteria invasion. The skin tries to protect the body from infection (being tagged). The germs are the infectious agents that sometimes get into the body causing illness. It can also be pointed out that as long as the skin remains intact, it wards off harmful disease agents and prevents infection from entering the body.

The second example shows how the game of Ball Pass Relay can be used to introduce the concept organs are groups of tissues working together to perform major functions of the body. Several circles are formed. The captain of each circle holds a ball. On a signal, the captain passes the ball to the right. The ball continues around the circle until it returns to the captain who immediately raises a hand. The team finishing first scores a point. Variations can be used such as (1) passing to the left, (2) passing the ball around the circle three or four times, (3) changing the type of passes, and (4) increasing the size of the circle to make passes longer.

In applying this game to the concept, the circles can be designated as the heart, lungs and other organs of the body. Each child can be compared to a tissue. Just as coordination and cooperation are necessary between the children in a circle to win the game, coordination and cooperation are necessary for tissues in order for organs to perform their functions. The variations in the game may suggest that, just as some of the skills are more difficult to perform than others, some of the functions of the organs of the body are more difficult to accomplish. But, with all of the tissues (and team members) working together, the difficult tasks can be accomplished.

The following simulated teaching-learning situation is presented to help point up the idea more clearly. The procedure shows how a second-grade teacher could use the active game of Run for Your Supper in a unit on foods.

Teacher: We sometimes hear people say that a healthy child is a hungry child. How many of you boys and girls run into the house quickly when your mother calls you to come in and eat?

Child: Sometimes I don't want to go in and eat because I have more fun playing.

Teacher: Yes, and I believe that is true of most children. However, we need to have strong muscles so that we can play. Because of this we need to eat certain kinds of foods, and perhaps we should eat at regular times. Now we are going outside, and I want to tell you about a new game we are going to play. The name of the game is Run for Your Supper. Why would this be a good game for us to learn just at this time?

Child: Because we are studying about food and how it makes you feel like playing if you eat right.

Teacher: Yes, that's right, and what does the name of this game make you think of?

Child: That you should hurry in to eat when you are called.

Child: That we need strong muscles to play, so kids should take time out to eat.

Teacher: Very good. George. An automobile would soon quit running if we didn't put gas in it, wouldn't it? Now, I am going to explain the game to you here in our room, and I want to see if you can remember how to play it when we get outside. We will form a circle and hold hands. One person will be chosen to be It. He or she will suddenly stop between two children and say, "Run for your supper!" Those two children will run in different directions around the circle. They will see which one of them can get back first to the place he or she left. The person to get back first can select It for the next time.

Child: This game is something like another one we played. I can't remember the name.

Teacher: Does anyone remember the name of that game?

Child: I think it was Slap Jack.

Teacher: Yes, that was it.

Child: I don't see how you do this.

Child: Neither do I.

Teacher: Very well, let's take a little time so some of you can show how we do it. Mary, Donald and Roy, come and stand in front of the room, please. Mary you be It and show us what happens.

Child: No, that won't work. They can't run if their hands are being held.

Child: How about if we put our hands on the two players' shoulders and said, "Run for Your Supper?" Everyone would know then that I was really It.

Teacher: I think that is a fine idea. Shall we try it that way? (The children proceed to the playground and participate in the game for a time; then the teacher evaluates it with them.)

Teacher: Shall we review some of the things we learned in the game, Run for Your Supper? Can someone tell us? Fred?

Child: We make a circle and It runs and chooses two to run. The next It is chosen by the last one back.

Teacher: Do you think the game Run for Your Supper will help you remember anything about what we are studying?

Child: Well, you should come in and eat when you are called instead of staying out to play some more.

Teacher: Can you give us one reason for that, Nancy?

Child: Well, then you will be able to play more, because you need food to be strong and play games.

Child: Good food helps make you strong, and maybe if you were hungry you would run faster.

Teacher: That might be. Can you think of ways we could make the game better?

Child: Try not to run into each other.

Teacher: Yes. Can you think of any way we could change the game so the players could have more turns?

Child: Couldn't we have more circles and have someone It for each one?

Teacher: That sounds like a good idea. Why don't we try that when we play a circle game again.

REASONS WHY CHILDREN LEARN THROUGH ACTIVE GAMES

During the early school years, and from ages six through eight particularly, learning can be limited frequently by a relatively short attention span rather than by intellectual capabilities alone. Moreover, some children who do not appear to think or learn well in abstract terms can more readily grasp concepts when given an opportunity to use them in an applied manner. In view of the fact that the young child lives in a movement world so to speak, and that he or she is likely to deal better in concrete rather than abstract terms, it would seem natural that the active-game medium is well suited for the development of certain concepts.

The above statement should not be interpreted as a suggestion that learning through movement-oriented experiences (motor learning) and passive learning experiences (verbal learning) are two different kinds of learning. The position is taken here that learning is learning, even though in the active-game approach the motor component may be operating at a higher level than in most of the traditional types of learning activities.

It is the premise here that problem-solving is an excellent way of human learning and that learning can take place well through problem-solving. In an active-game learning situation that is well planned, a great deal of consideration is given to the inherent possibilities for learning in terms of problem-solving. In fact, in most active games, opportunities abound for near-ideal teaching-learning situations because there are many problems to be solved.

Another very important consideration with respect to the nature of learning through active games is that a considerable numbers of the learnings of young children are motor in character, the child devoting a good proportion of his or her attention to skills of a locomotor nature. Furthermore, learnings of a motor nature tend to usurp a large amount of the young child's time and energy, and are often closely associated with other learnings. In addition, it is well known by experienced K-3 grade teachers that the child's motor mechanism is active to the extent that it is almost impossible to remain quiet for very long, regardless of the passiveness of the learning situation.

Some of the general aspects of the value of the active-game learning medium have been presented. The discussion that follows will focus more specifically upon certain inherent facilitative factors in active games that are highly compatible with children's learning. These factors are (1) motivation, (2) proprioception, and (3) reinforcement, all of which are somewhat interdependent and interrelated.

MOTIVATION

In general, the child is motivated when he or she discovers what seems to be a suitable reason for engaging in a certain activity. The most valid reason, of course, is that the child sees a purpose for the activity and derives enjoyment from it. The child must feel that what is being done is important and purposeful. When this occurs and the child gets the impression of success in a group situation, motivation comes about naturally as a result of his or her concern for the activity. It is the premise here that the active-game approach contains this built in ingredient so necessary to desirable and worthwhile learning.

As far as active games are concerned, we need to consider motivation in terms of (1) interest, (2) knowledge of results, and (3) competition.

With regard to interest there is a principle of learning that suggests that learning is likely to be enhanced when the child agrees with and acts upon the learnings considered of most value. This means that the child accepts as most valuable those things that are of greatest interest. To most children, their active play experiences are of the greatest personal value to them.

Under most circumstances a very high interest level is concomitant with active-game situations simply because of the expectation of pleasure children tend to associate with such activities. The structure of a learning activity is directly related to the length of time the learning act can be tolerated by the learner without loss of interest. Active-game situations by their very nature are more likely to hold the children's attention than many of the traditional learning activities.

Considering motivation from the point of view of knowledge of results, the active-game approach to learning provides almost instantaneous knowledge of results because the child can actually see and feel throwing a ball, tagging or being tagged in a game. He or she does not become the victim of a poorly-constructed paper and pencil test, the results of which may have little or no meaning for the child. This is particularly important as far as some slower-learning children are concerned.

In commenting on competition as a factor of motivation, it might be well to repeat the description of active games that appeared at the outset of the chapter; that is, active games imply active interactions of children in cooperative and/or competitive situations. It is possible to have both cooperation and competition functioning at the same time, as in the case of team games. While one team is competing against the other, there is cooperation within each team. It is also possible to have one group competing against another without cooperation within the groups.

It is interesting to note that the terms cooperation and competition are opposite in meaning; therefore, the reconciliation of children's competitive needs and cooperative needs is not an easy matter. In a sense we are confronted with an ambivalent condition which, if not carefully handled, could place children in a state of conflict. Modern society not only rewards one kind of behavior (competition), but its direct opposite (cooperation). Perhaps more often than not our cultural demands sanction these rewards without providing clear-cut standards of value regarding specific conditions under which these forms of behavior might be practiced. Thus, the child is placed in somewhat of a quandary with reference to when to compete and when to cooperate. As far as active games are concerned, they not only appear to be a good medium for learning because of the intrinsic motivation inherent in them, but also this medium of learning can provide the competition children need in a pleasurable and enjoyable way.

PROPRIOCEPTION

Generally speaking, proprioception is concerned with muscle sense. The proprioceptors are sensory nerve terminals that give information concerning movements and position of the body. A proprioceptive feedback mechanism is involved which, in a sense, regulates movement. In view of the fact that children are movement-oriented, it appears a reasonable speculation that proprioceptive feedback from the receptors of muscles, skin and joints contributes in a facilitative manner when the active-game medium is used to develop academic skills and concepts.

REINFORCEMENT

In considering the compatibility of the active-game learning medium with reinforcement theory, the meaning of reinforcement needs to be taken into account. An acceptable general description of reinforcement would be that the increase in the efficiency of a response to a stimulus is brought about by the concurrent action of another stimulus. The basis for contending that the active-game learning medium is consistent with general reinforcement theory is that this medium reinforces attention to the learning task and learning behavior. It keeps children involved in the learning activity which is perhaps the major area of application for reinforcement procedures. Moreover, there is perhaps little in the way of human behavior that is not reinforced or at least reinforcible by feedback of some sort, and the importance of proprioceptive feedback has already been mentioned in this particular connection.

ACTIVE GAMES INVOLVING HEALTH CONCEPTS

It has been suggested throughout the chapter that there are a number of health concepts that might be developed by children as they engage in certain active games. Moreover, some examples of some of these possibilities have been given. As in the case of any kind of learning situation, it should not be expected that these concepts will develop automatically. Skillful teacher guidance is needed, and when the teacher knows that a concept is more or less inherent in a given activity, there is a better chance that he or she will make a concentrated effort to develop the concept. The active games suggested here that contain inherent health concepts have been used with success by elementary school teachers. Descriptions of the activities follow the summary of them. In some cases, specific applications for the games are suggested. In others, just the game and concept are given and it is suggested that the reader work out his or her own application.

Game	Topic	Concept
Germ and Toothbrush	Dental Health	One of the ways of preventing tooth decay is brushing the teeth soon after eating.
Hot Potato	Body Function	Our brain sends us messages to tell us to react quickly, protecting us from danger.
Circle Pass Ball	Disease	Cold germs are spread by direct contact. One way of preventing colds is to keep away from others when you have a cold.
Change Circle Relay	Food	A balanced diet is good for health.
Ball Pass	Body Function	The circulation of the blood through the body helps the blood perform many functions.

Policeman	Pedestrian Safety	There are many devices used as a means of safety, one of which is the traffic light.
Cross the Street	Pedestrian Safety	We should always look up and down the street before crossing to make sure no cars are coming.
Fire in the House	Fire Prevention	Fires can be harmful and destructive and we must guard against this.
Fruit Basket	Food	We should eat certain foods to grow strong and healthy.
Hill Dill	Exercise and Playground Safety	Outdoor play is important to good health (exercise). Always watch where you are going in a running and tag game (playground safety).
Attention	Body Mechanics	Erect posture is important in daily living. A strong, well-balanced framework can assume different positions. Muscles along the framework hold the body in good balance with little effort.

GERM AND TOOTHBRUSH

One of the ways of preventing tooth decay is brushing the teeth soon after eating. About ten to twelve players join hands in a semicircle. Another player hides behind these players and is the one who flees. Another player stands in the middle of the semicircle, shuts the eyes and counts to ten. This player then tries to find the one hiding and gives chase. The players in the semicircle let the chaser in and out as he or she chooses, but try to keep out the one being chased. The game can continue until the one chased is caught or a new chaser is named. The children who are standing in the semicircle holding hands are the teeth in the mouth. The chaser is the toothbrush. The other player, the one hiding and fleeing, is the germ. The toothbrush tries to catch the germ hiding in the mouth. The teeth help the toothbrush.

HOT POTATO

Our brain sends us messages to tell us to react quickly, protecting us from danger. All players stand in a circle formation. A ball or beanbag is passed rapidly from player to player around the circle. Following it are three or four other balls or beanbags, each starting at a different place in the circle. If an object is dropped a point is scored against that player. At a signal, all passing stops instantly, and those holding an object have a point scored against them; the game then continues as before. A winner is determined by the lowest score after a specified playing time. The objects passed are considered to be very hot. Imagination must be used to recognize this fact. Since our brain tells us that an object is hot and painful, we get rid of the pain-causing element. The game illustrates this when the ball or beanbag is passed to the next person. Children acquire a fast reaction to something hot. They can understand how quickly our brain informs us of danger or other messages, and act accordingly to these messages.

CIRCLE PASS BALL

Cold germs are spread by direct contact. One way of preventing spread of colds is to keep away from others when you have a cold. Any number of children form a single circle facing inward. There should be a space of about three feet between players. The teacher or one child chosen to be the leader stands in the center. A ball is thrown quickly from one player to another around the circle. The teacher or child who is the leader gives a signal, and the child having the ball at that time has a point scored against him or her. This child goes to the center of the circle and the game continues. In this game, the ball represents the cold germ. The idea is to pass the ball as soon as possible so as not to be caught with the germ.

CHANGE CIRCLE RELAY

A balanced diet is good for health. The children make rows behind a starting line in teams of four each. About 30 feet in front of each team there are two circles drawn touching each other. In one of the circles, three ten pins or other suitable objects are placed. On a signal, the first child on each team runs up to the circles and removes the pins from the first to the second circle, and then returns to the rear of the team. The second child then runs up and puts the pins back in the first circle and returns in the same manner. The first team to finish is the winner. The four members of each team represent the four food groups, and, if desired, can be so named. It can be pointed out that a well-balanced diet needs all four food groups, and these four groups can work together to make a person healthy. The teacher can help the children see that just as all the children on a team are needed to make it a winning team, a balanced diet is essential for good health, and every type of food is important.

BALL PASS

The circulation of the blood through the body helps the blood perform many functions. The children form a circle and pass a rubber ball around the circle to a rhythmic pattern. The first pattern could be bounce-catch-bounce-catch, and the next could be bounce-bounce-bounce-catch. With two balls in play, a continuous pattern is established. The children must be alert and ready for the oncoming ball. The first child bounces the ball to the second child; the second child catches it and bounces it on to the next child. As the second ball is put into play, the first child bounces the ball three times and, on the third bounce, sends it on to the next child. That child catches the ball and repeats the process. The balls are thought of as the blood, and the players represent the blood vessels which carry the blood to all members or parts of the body which is the entire group. When the balls make a complete circle, the children keep the ball going because blood circulates over and over. The children can be helped to understand that keeping the balls in a rhythmic pattern is like the pulse beat when they learn to locate the pulse in the temple, throat and wrists.

POLICEMAN

There are many devices used as a means of safety, one of which is the traffic light. One child is selected to be the policeman, and sides are chosen. The sides stand equidistant from the policeman. The policeman carries a card, red on one side and green on the other. At the signal to go (green) from the policeman, each side sees how far it can get before the stop signal (red) is given. Any child who moves after the signal is given must go back to the original starting point. When all members of a side have passed the policeman, that side is declared the winner.

CROSS THE STREET

We should always look up and down the street before crossing to make sure no cars are coming. The class is divided into two equal groups. An area is designated as the street and lines are drawn to indicate the width and length of the street. One group lines up on one side of the street and the other group lines up on the other side. One player on each side is selected to be a vehicle. The vehicles take their places at each end of the street rather than at the sides of the street. On a signal from the teacher the vehicles begin to move from either end of the street. The players on the sides of the street must cross before the vehicles reach the opposite ends. All players who come close enough to the vehicles to be tagged or fail to reach the other side of the street in time have a point scored against their side. The group with the least number of points scored against it is the winner.

FIRE IN THE HOUSE

Fire can be harmful and destructive and we must guard against this. The players form a circle, facing the center. A ball representing fire is given to one of the players. Another ball of a different size or color, representing the house, is given to another player approximately one-third of the way around the circle from the player with the first ball. On a signal from the teacher, the players begin to hand the fire and the house around the circle from one player to another. The idea of the game is to try to catch the house with the fire, and, at the same time, to keep the fire from catching the house. The teacher may give a signal at certain times for the game to stop. When the game stops, a point is scored against the children who have possession of either ball. The game continues in this manner for a specified playing time.

FRUIT BASKET

We should eat certain foods to grow strong and healthy. Fruit Basket is played by children forming a circle, facing the center. One player is designated as the caller and stands in the center of the circle. The players in the circle are given the names of different kinds of fruit. To start the game, the caller calls out the names of two kinds of fruit. The players with these two names attempt to change places, while the caller tries to tag one of them. The caller may call out, "Upset the fruit basket." When this call is given, everyone must change to a different position. The game continues, with several children being given the opportunity to be the caller.

HILL DILL

Outdoor play is important to good health (exercise). Always watch where you are going in a running and tag game. Two parallel goal lines are established approximately 60 feet apart. One person is selected to be It and stands midway between the two goal lines. The rest of the class is divided into two equal groups, one group standing on one goal line and the other on the other goal line. It calls out, "Hill, dill, run over the hill." At this signal, the players on each of the goal lines run to the other goal line. It tries to tag as many as possible while they are exchanging goals. All of those tagged become helpers and the game continues in this manner until all but one have been tagged. This person is It for the next game.

ATTENTION

Erect posture is important in daily living. A strong, well-balanced framework can assume different positions. Muscles along the framework hold the body in good balance with little effort. This game is played by dividing the class into four equal groups. The members of each group stand side-by-side to form a line. The four lines form in such a manner that they make a square. The corners of the square should be open so that there is plenty of running space. The members of each line are numbered consecutively from left to right so that each person in the line has a different number. However, there will be four persons with the same number, one from each line. The teacher or a child selected as the leader calls out a number, and all four persons having that number run around their own line and back to their original position. The first one back scores five points for the team; the second, three points; and the third, one point. The game continues in this manner for a specified period of time. All groups come to attention before each signal is given to run. When the signal is given, the others stand in a rest position.

SUGGESTIONS FOR SUPPLEMENTARY READING

Blum, H.T. and Yocum, D.J., A fun alternative: using instructional games to foster student learning, *Teaching Exceptional Children*, 29, November/December 1996, p. 60-3.

Butler, J.I., Teacher responses to teaching games for understanding, *Journal of Physical Education, Recreation, and Dance*, 67, November/December 1996, p. 17-20.

Conkell, C.S. and Pearson, H., Do you use developmentally appropriate games? *Strategies*, 9, September 1995, p. 22-5.

Curtner-Smith, M.D., Teaching for understanding using games invention with elementary children, *Journal of Physical Education, Recreation and Dance*, 67, March 1996, p. 33-7.

Dominick, A. and Clark, F.B., Using games to understand children's understanding, *Childhood Education*, 72 (annual theme issue) 1996, p. 286-8.

Grambo, G., The games that kids play, *Gifted Child Today Magazine*, 18, September/October, p. 17.

Griffin, L.L., et al., Pedagogical content knowledge for teachers, *Journal of Physical Education, Recreation and Dance*, 67, November/December 1996, p. 58-61.

Humphrey, J.H., *Integration of Physical Education in the Elementary School Curriculum*, Springfield, IL, Charles C Thomas Publisher, 1990, p. 56-67.

Lehwald, H.D. and Greene, L., Game adaptation: essential to health integration with physical education, *The Physical Educator*, 53, Spring 1996, p. 94-101.

Ragon, B.M. and Bennett, J.P., Something more to consider: combining health education and physical education, *Journal of Physical Education, Recreation and Dance*, 67, January 1996, p. 14-15.

CHAPTER 11

INTEGRATION OF HEALTH AND CREATIVE EXPRESSION

Childhood and creativity go together. Young children are naturally creative. They have vivid imaginations. They pretend. They enjoy "make believe". They are original and ingenious in their thoughts and actions. They ask questions. They want to know "why". Their thoughts can soar to heights unknown. To the elementary school child the world is full of adventure, excitement, and wonder. Each child is born with, and therefore, possesses, intellectual ability-unknown in quantity and quality.

Children differ widely in their interests, abilities, and needs. Thus, the elementary school curriculum should be designed to provide a balance of daily experiences through which the child might find varied and appropriate opportunities to express himself or herself creatively. It is assumed that there is a place for creativity in all school subjects. No longer is creative expression thought of only in such areas as art, music, writing and dramatics. More and more the value of creativity is recognized in areas of learning that were formerly thought of as being rather routine. Through the nurture of the individual's creative ability, he or she can be guided to the threshold of new ideas and discoveries in such areas as health, mathematics, language arts, science, social studies, and physical education.

Creative thinking is based essentially upon the *concepts learned through experience*. It should follow that the richer the concept, the more possibilities for its expression. It is suggested that the essence of creativity lies in (1) an abundance and wealth of ideas; (2) thoughts and feelings to express; and (3) a variety of media for expression. In other words, creative expression to be effective might well be integrated with the whole program of instruction. Creativity tends to clarify, stimulate, and extend the child's learnings and, thereby, causes the individual to operate at higher levels of ability and with wider ranges of competency.

Creative expression should enable the teacher to gain insight into what the child thinks and feels. Guided self-expression can offer children appropriate releases for inner tensions, and at the same time enable them to add stature to their feelings of worth. Freedom to be creative tends to make children happier, more relaxed, more productive, more purposeful, and mature in all aspects of their total health. The creative teacher exercises skill by (1) recognizing and accepting ideas of each child; (2) guiding and channeling, but not controlling, the development of the child's ideas; and (3) assisting the child to bring ideas to fruition; and (4) enabling the child to present ideas to others. Through such procedures, creative activities can have a kind of therapeutic value. This approach constitutes one very effective way of reaching all children.

HEALTH AND CREATIVE EXPRESSION

Children probably use language for creative expression more than any other medium. A child tends to feel a need for an adequate vocabulary of appropriate words to express thoughts and feelings clearly and in a form that conveys the precise meanings to others.

Some children who do not express themselves well in oral or written communication may do well in other media. Creative expression can appear in many different forms and through many different media such as the extension of one's self through expression in art, music, and dramatics. It is becoming recognized more and more that art, music, and dramatics have a vast potential contribution to make to the total health of the individual. An educational program that includes experiences in these areas should help children to:

Discover and develop special aptitudes and talents

Express themselves creatively

Communicate feelings in a creative and aesthetic manner

Understand and appreciate their environment

Develop emotional stability by releasing tension
Develop self-confidence and self-control
Enjoy the finer aspects of life
Use leisure time more wisely
Develop social relationships among children of similar interest
Enrich other areas of learning

HEALTH AND CREATIVE ART ACTIVITIES

For many years art has been considered an important part of the elementary school program. It is a very natural means of expression for the young child. With whatever materials are available an elementary school child rather intuitively will spend his or her own time manipulating and experimenting to find ways of expression. Consequently, during the elementary school years the major emphasis is on a basic art program, that makes it possible for children to have experiences with a large variety of materials, rather than on a meager program limited to the use of a few materials.

Art in the elementary school should perhaps be creative and exploratory. One of its unique contributions lies in providing first-hand experience with various processes involving the use of numerous materials. The resourceful teacher knows that the first step toward a successful art program for children is the availability of numerous materials to care for their individual needs, aptitudes, and interests. As in other areas of learning, a child may have a particular aptitude for one facet of art rather than another. In other words, a child who finds little satisfaction in painting scenery for a health play, may be especially adept at sawing, cutting, nailing, making holes, and finishing a fence for a garden scene in the same play.

Creative art experiences need skillful guidance by the teacher, from the stimulation of ideas to the finishing of the product. A knowledge of the creative process takes on added significance as the teacher provides numerous opportunities for the children to learn the use of the various art media. These experiences usually follow a somewhat planned sequence, as follows:

1. There is a manipulative stage when the child becomes acquainted with the art media. The child learns the names of the materials and tools. He or she handles them, and discusses their use and care.

2. There is an experimental stage when the child learns firsthand how to use the material or tool to create colors, forms, balance, contrast, emphasis, and lines. He or she learns from the experiences of experimenting, without the pressure of having to produce something acceptable.

3. There is an expressive or productive state when the child selects and uses certain media to express thoughts and feelings.

It should be remembered that in all art activities, the emphasis should be upon the total development of the child as well as upon the mastery of skills and techniques. Creative art activities can contribute to the total health of the individual. On the other hand, health teaching provides opportunities for self-expression through art. The examples given here indicate a few of the ways creative teachers might attempt to integrate the use of some of the various art materials and tools to further health teaching.

COLOR MEDIA

Crayons, colored chalk, finger paints, water colors, tempura paints, and charcoal are some of the media that may be used in art activities to summarize and record health concepts. Spatter, stencil, and sponge painting provide variations and interest to the work with colors.

HEALTH ACTIVITIES INVOLVING COLOR MEDIA

Make a colored drawing showing circulatory system, or other systems of the body.

Color a series of original pictures showing how germs are transmitted.

Make a charcoal drawing to show ways to avoid fires.

Color original pictures for a calendar showing safety practices for each month of the year.

Color place mats for the teachers in the building. Use spatter, stencil, or sponge paintings.

Color scenery for a health play, "Vacation Fun."

Design prints for dress or shirt material.

THREE-DIMENSIONAL CONSTRUCTION

The tools and materials used in three-dimensional construction provide for common groups interests as children give expression to their feelings through creative endeavors. Construction might include the making of such items as:

1. Dioramas (panoramic scenes constructed for depicting activities related to health).
2. Relief maps of areas showing physical features.
3. Mobiles (a number of shapes usually suspended from a wire frame and moving freely in space).
4. Stabiles (a number of shapes usually attached to a stationary base).
5. Miniature buildings and equipment.

HEALTH ACTIVITIES INVOLVING THREE-DIMENSIONAL CONSTRUCTION

Make a diorama to show what constitutes a desirable picnic area.

Make a diorama to show the natural habitat of fur-bearing animals that supply raw materials for clothing.

Make a diorama to show safety in water sports.

Make mobiles to show what constitutes a good breakfast.

Make mobiles to show items needed for good grooming.

Construct a relief map to show well-known vacation areas in the United States. Use pipe-cleaner figures to identify the sports-skiing in Vermont, water sports in Florida.

Construct a relief map to show areas that produce raw materials for clothes.

Construct a grocery store with shelves, counters, refrigerators, and so on.

Construct equipment used in a bakery, such as a mixer, weighing machine, bread troughs, ovens.

Construct a miniature dairy farm with buildings.

CREATIVE CRAFTS

Carving, modeling, weaving, making toys and games, costuming, pipe-cleaner crafts, and papier-maché puppets and masks furnish media for children to use in connection with their study of health.

HEALTH ACTIVITIES INVOLVING CREATIVE CRAFTS

Make a bat stand and bags for the bases in softball.

Make bean bags.

Make picture puzzles.

Make toys such as kites and airplanes.

Weave paper place mats for a party at school to enjoy products of milk.

Make soap carvings of the different kinds of seafood.

Make papier-maché masks for a play about animals that give us raw materials for clothing.

Mold items such as meats, fruits, vegetables, milk products and bakery items to be used in the classroom's grocery store.

Make pipe-cleaner dolls to illustrate safety in and near the water.

Make costumes for the children in a health play on the story of bread.

Make life-size cardboard figures for a display window in the classroom. Dress the figures for different summertime activities, such as parties, picnics, and swimming.

LETTERING

Lettering aids children to label and identify health materials for exhibits, displays, bulletin boards, charts, and booklets. Block and stick printing can be used for decorative purposes also.

HEALTH ACTIVITIES INVOLVING PRINTING

Make and label a health picture for younger children.

Make a chart showing good manners when eating.

Make picture charts showing a good breakfast, lunch, and dinner.

Cut block prints to use for making get-well cards.

Make and label a pictorial chart of the four food groups.

Make and label a chart showing various types of bread.

Make a pictorial calendar for the vegetable garden. Record planting dates, growth of plants, and harvesting of vegetables.

Make a chart indicating the child responsible for each duty involved in vegetable gardening.

Make a booklet of types of tools used for the vegetable garden.

Make posters of safety rules for the school grounds.

Make and label a display of resources used to produce synthetic materials.

Make an exhibit of foods containing the various vitamins.

Make a poster of the vegetable seeds planted in the garden. Attach the package container for each kind of seed.

Letter appropriate captions for a bulletin board centered around good manners in the cafeteria.

Use stick prints to decorate a paper tablecloth and napkins for breakfast in the classroom.

Compile a book of simple recipes that include milk.

Arrange a central hall bulletin board and display case for special health drives, such as, Junior Red Cross, Dental Health Week, Easter Seals for Crippled Children and the like.

MURALS AND FRIEZES

For purposes of this discussion a mural will refer to a wall decoration with one specific theme, while a frieze will mean a wall decoration composed of a series of related themes.

HEALTH ACTIVITIES INVOLVING MURALS AND FRIEZES

Make a mural to show poisonous plants in the community.

Make a mural to show foods that help us to have good teeth.

Make a mural to show ways to rest and relax.

Make a mural to show the different kinds of fruits.

Make a series of murals to show various ways fruits are processed.

Make a mural to show milk products.

Make a frieze to show the story of cotton from the seed to our clothes.

Make a frieze to show the story of milk from the cow to the table.

Make a frieze to show the story of bread; include planting the grain, threshing the grain, grinding the grain, making bread, wrapping bread, and delivering bread.

Make a frieze to show health services available at the health center.

HEALTH AND CREATIVE MUSIC ACTIVITIES

Music is considered a very important part of the curriculum offerings in the elementary school. From the beginning of formal education, the child should experience the joys that come from participating in each facet of the total music program; that is (1) singing, (2) music appreciation, (3) instrumental music, and (4) creative music. Each facet has a potential unique contribution to make to the total health of the individual.

Music offers avenues for creative expression at all levels of the elementary school. Rather frequently, children at play can be observed humming an original tune, singing a familiar couplet to music of their own, or trying a new step to music they enjoy. Indeed, it appears that music holds a unique fascination for most children. The resourceful teacher can capitalize upon the child's desire for self-expression through music as a means of furthering growth and development-emotionally, socially, physically, and intellectually, as well as furthering his or her knowledge in the various aspects of total health

Health offers innumerable opportunities for creative activities in music. The activities suggested below are intended as illustrations of ways that health can be integrated with creative expression in such areas as singing, music appreciation and instrumental music.

HEALTH AND CREATIVE SINGING

Experience has shown in many cases that children delight in singing original tunes in answer to health questions asked by the teacher. For example, the teacher could sing: "How did you brush your teeth today?" The child sings his or her own tune and words in response. Or, the teacher might sing:

When should you wash your hands?

When do you need to take a bath?

How do you feel about losing a ball game?

What do you do to get ready for breakfast?

Why do you like to drink milk?

Children sing their own tunes and words in response.

Children have been known to create health songs – sometimes the music as well as the lyrics – but more frequently they write words for familiar tunes. The classic example is probably the music for "Here We Go Round The Mulberry Bush". To this melody the children add their own words and actions, such as:

This is the way we wash our hands,

Wash our hands,

Wash our hands,

This is the way we skip to school,

Skip to school,

Skip to school.

Creative songs have a freshness and charm of their own. This aspect of creativity needs stimulation, encouragement, and recognition, for its value lies in what happens to the child once he or she finds another avenue for expression and enjoyment.

HEALTH AND MUSIC APPRECIATION

Probably words can never express the intangible associated with the aesthetic values one can derive from listening to good music. Few would dispute its value in terms of its contributions to one's health. The teacher's attitude toward music is extremely important. It is the teacher who has the responsibility for creating an atmosphere in which there is the time to listen to music, simply for the joy of listening. In such an atmosphere, children may want to discuss what they hear and how they feel, or they may want to express their thoughts and feelings through other media. Sometimes, it is enough simply to want to listen again.

HEALTH AND CREATIVE INSTRUMENTAL MUSIC

Children like to create sounds and music. They may pick out a tune on the piano; they may create a tune on whatever instrument is at hand. Elementary school children can make simple instrument on which to create music. They can tune water glasses, carve willow whistles, and make rhythmic instruments such as bells, cymbals, drums, maracas, rattles, rhythm sticks, sandblocks, tambourines, and triangles. In singing, the child uses the voice to create sounds and tunes, and in this facet of music, he or she needs opportunities to create sounds and music with instruments.

Health offers many activities with which creative instrumental music can be integrated. For example, during periods of relaxation, children can move around the classroom to the varying tempo produced on the homemade instruments. Children can rest at their desks to the soft music played on tuned water glasses. Summarizing activities to health units can be enhanced by original instrumentation worked out to add atmosphere to the presentation.

HEALTH AND CREATIVE DRAMATICS

Through the ages, creative expression through dramatics has been an effective means used to communicate our thoughts and feelings to others. As with other media of creativity, dramatics can contribute to the total health of the individual. It is through dramatics that children can (1) release or greatly reduce tensions and fears; (2) resolve real and imaginary problems in a satisfactory manner; (3) develop feelings of empathy based on deeper understandings; (4) build sound patterns of behavior; (5) learn to express themselves well through speech, gestures, and bodily movement; and (6) develop feelings of security, adequacy and belongingness while sharing common experiences with their peers.

Creative dramatic experiences involve (1) dramatic play, (2) pantomime, (3) informal dramatization, (4) puppetry, and (5) formal dramatizations. Dramatics, as a creative approach to learning, is especially adaptable to health teaching. The remainder of this chapter will deal with various suggestions for the integration of health and creative expression through dramatics.

HEALTH AND DRAMATIC PLAY

Dramatic play characterizes the spontaneous, undirected activities in which children engage during early childhood, including kindergarten and first grade. Through dramatic play, children make believe they are adults, and live through the adult life they see going on around them. They identify themselves with people by playing the role of mother, father, teacher, relatives, milkman, grocer and the like.

Role playing provides a creative approach to learning. Among other things, it makes language development purposeful, and at the same time it can reveal the child – his or her talents and abilities as well as fears and misinterpretations – to the teacher. The major emphasis in dramatic play is upon the role. For the most part, children volunteer for the role they want to play. In so doing, it is important that the child assume the role and identify with it to the extent that he or she expresses the feelings involved without inhibitions.

Dramatic play in health offers as many possibilities as there are roles to play in a given lesson or unit. For instance, children might role-play:

The school nurse explaining to the children about how to prevent common colds

The dentist examining teeth

Mother preparing a meal

Mother shopping at a supermarket

Father helping the children get ready for bed

Mother buying school clothes for the children

Big sister setting the dinner table

The policeman directing traffic at street crossing nearest the school

Under teacher guidance, the children can show the teacher what they have learned in health by selecting the characters they want to portray, and creating the dialogue and actions. Usually children want to repeat the "play". In so doing, they change their roles and much of the dialogue each time the roles are played.

HEALTH AND PANTOMIME

Through pantomime, a child expresses thoughts and feelings by the use of facial expressions, gestures, and movements without speaking. Any lines to be spoken, read, or sung are done by others than the child doing the acting. Since pantomime requires only physical expressions, it has real value for the shy, timid child who will act a part that requires no talking. This applies equally well to the child with a speech defect or impediment. As valuable as it may be as a means of expression for certain children, it should be understood that pantomime constitutes one important part of the creative dramatic experience for all children.

HEALTH AND INFORMAL DRAMATIZATION

Dramatic play and pantomime represent activities that are adapted to the growth and development of the young child, who is still self-centered, and normally plays as an individual even when among other children. As the child begins to relate to others, he or she is ready for a type of dramatization that involves interaction with groups of children. Therefore, informal dramatization comes after the child has had some experiences with dramatic play and pantomime. Informal dramatization is characterized by its spontaneity, naturalness of expression, and simplicity of organization. Very little if anything is needed in the way of stage and properties. The child's imagination seems to fill the gap. For instance, a chair can serve as the dining-room table in one informal dramatization, and the same chair can be a washbowl in the next play. To the child, the "play's the thing." It is self-sustaining and self-sufficient.

Among other things, informal dramatization develops creativity, originality, imagination and fluency of speech among children. It can aid also in the development of social understandings. Through sociodrama, or informal dramatization based upon a social problem, the children can express their own feelings directly or indirectly toward a problem. In this manner he or she learns how to meet the problem by trying different solutions and observing the consequences. For instance, there could be such problems as: How late should children be permitted to watch television on a school night? Should all children in the home be treated alike? How can a child, who is a leader most of the time, become a good follower in the group? Through informal, unrehearsed dramatizations of problems similar to these, the child gains insights and a different perspective in terms of what seem to be possible best solutions. In sociodrama, the emphasis is upon the social problem or situation, whereas, in role-playing the emphasis is on the role.

Another aspect of informal dramatization is psychodrama. However, since psychodrama deals with emotional problems that the child is experiencing, it is usually handled in private and by a specialist in mental health.

HEALTH AND PUPPETRY

Puppets serve as players in carrying out dramatic interpretations. Since children identify puppets with human beings, puppets can be used to help children develop positive and objective understandings relating to the lives of others. The use of puppets can stimulate creativeness, individuality, inventiveness, and originality on the part of those involved. The effectiveness of a production depends upon the manipulation of the puppets, and the use of the voice to carry the mood and intent and to portray vividly the feelings to be communicated.

Puppets serve as another means which the teacher might use to reach the shy, withdrawn, or self-conscious child, who refrains from appearing before an audience. Since the necessity for personal appearance is eliminated, the child who finds other audience situations difficult may do quite well concealed behind the puppet stage. Children with speech impediments have been known to speak fluently and distinctly in a puppet show once they have identified themselves with the puppets.

Puppets offer a variety of possibilities for health teaching. One procedure which has been successful is that in which puppets have been used to introduce a health unit. This procedure is particularly effective with K-3 level children, because it tends to hold their interest while a new topic is being initiated. Puppets are suitable at any grade level, and constitute an essential part of a balanced program in dramatics for the elementary school child.

HEALTH AND FORMAL DRAMATIZATION

Formal dramatization differs from other forms of dramatics in that it necessitates more thorough planning of the plot, characterizations, dialogue, staging, and costumes. On the other hand, formal dramatizations relating to health contain elements of the other forms of creative dramatics: that is, (1) the enacting of a role (role-playing); (2) the use of facial expressions, gestures, and movements (pantomime); (3) the emphasis on a social problem or situation (informal dramatization); (4) the use of the voice to carry the intent and mood, and to portray feelings to be communicated (puppetry); and (5) staging and costuming (puppetry). Moreover, formal dramatization provides highly motivated, functional situations for improving the language arts skills, from the decision to write a health play to the final curtain at the end of the production. Therefore, it is extremely important that the purposes for a formal dramatization be clearly defined in terms of inherent learning experiences rather than as an extravaganza for the entertainment of an audience.

Formal dramatization can utilize creativeness in (1) writing the play; (2) varying the dialogues and actions; (3) producing simple costumes and staging; and (4) working out personal interpretations, as children release themselves to become the character they are portraying.

HEALTH PLAYS

If used wisely health plays may serve as a satisfactory supplement to the health learning situation. There are two general sources of health plays: those that are developed by the children themselves and those that are published by official and voluntary health agencies, and by some commercial groups. Health plays devised by children under the guidance of the teacher have more merit in that they draw upon the creative ability of children who have a special aptitude for this type of activity.

Experimentation with health plays indicates that this type of activity has two rather specific applications. One is that a health play may be used in the form of an introductory activity. The teacher may employ this approach by selecting and working with a few class members prior to the time a health unit is introduced. Experience has shown that the genuine enthusiasm of children for play activity enhances its potentiality as an approach to the unit. A second way concerns how a health play may be used as part of a teaching unit in the form of an evaluation technique. Children can create a health play in order to dramatize those things that were learned in the study of the health unit. This procedure is of particular importance in the evaluation of health attitudes.

SUGGESTIONS FOR SUPPLEMENTARY READING

Burton, D., Engaging children in conversation about art, 96, *School Arts*, January 1997, p. 6.

Cline, D.B., and Ingerson, D., The mystery of Humpty's fall: primary-school children as playmakers, *Young Children*, 51, September 1996, p. 4-10.

Hargreaves, D.J., Teachers' assessments of primary children's classroom work in the creative arts, *Educational Research*, 38, Summer 1996, p. 199-211.

Jalongo, J.R., Using recorded music with young children: a guide for nonmusicians, *Young Children*, 51, July 1996, p. 6-14.

Jones, J.E., Make-believe makes sense, *Learning*, 24, May/June 1996, p. 36-7.

Killian, J.N., Definitions of "knowing": comparison of verbal report versus performance of children's songs, *Journal of Research in Music Education*, 44, Fall 1996, p. 215-28.

Kolb, G.R., Read with a beat: developing literacy through music and song, 50, *The Reading Teacher*, 50, September 1996, p. 76-7.

Lindquist, T., Use simple puppets to connect core subjects, *Instructor*, 106, August 1996, p. 91-2.

O'Day, S., Creative drama engages children's imaginations, *Gifted Child Today Magazine*, 19, September/October 1996, p. 16-19.

Westberg, K.L., The effects of teaching students how to invent, *The Journal of Creative Behavior*, 30, April 1996, p. 249-67.

CHAPTER 12

SCHOOL HEALTH EVALUATION

In Chapter 4 evaluation was discussed in terms of its place in the individual teaching-learning situation. The discussion in this final chapter considers the broader view of evaluation as it is applied to the entire school health program.

The term *evaluation* derived from the French word *evaluer* means, in a purely literal sense, to estimate or place a value on. When applied to health education, evaluation is considered as a more or less scientific way of determining the extent to which objectives of health education are being accomplished. In other words, evaluation in health education proposes to place a value on the outcomes which might be expected as a result of working with children in matters which presently, and in the future, may concern their health. Thus, measures need to be taken to determine the extent to which these outcomes are reached. In this connection, it appears important as a preface to subsequent discussions to differentiate between the terms *measurement* and *evaluation*.

Evaluation can be made with respect to three different aspects as follows:

1. Evaluation made with reference to the objectives one is attempting to achieve, establishing criteria of behavior expected of the child.

2. Evaluation made with regard to collection of *data* to determine what is happening to the child and the extent of desired behavioral changes.

3. Evaluation made in terms of the *significance* of the data collected, the interpretation of the data and the action to take as a result of the data.

The term *measurement* will likely be primarily confined to the second item above. Measurement is concerned with the quantitative aspect, and accurate data must be collected in order to arrive at a valid measurement. It is partly because of this that evaluation in the area of health education is a difficult matter. While accurate measurement may help provide a better means of evaluation, in health education it may not always be possible to rely entirely upon it. Thus, because of its many facets and ramifications, it may be necessary to use many evaluative techniques, subjective as well as objective, in the area of health education.

The process of evaluation is continuous, and consideration should be given to the data at every step of program development. Evaluation should not be considered solely as a terminal procedure, but cyclical, involving assessment, development, implementation and evaluation. Before curriculum writing begins, an assessment should be made of the health needs of the children and community. During the program, the continuous evaluation provides feedback that may prompt curricular or method changes. Upon completion of a program, a more complete assessment will prove valuable, providing input for change or reinforcement for an innovative technique. Repeating this procedure is more likely to result in a better program.

PURPOSES OF EVALUATION

Some of the purposes of the evaluation of the school health program are (1) to assess health needs and interests of (a) individuals, (b) groups and (c) the school-related community; (2) to assess the strengths and weaknesses of the total program including assessment of the components of the school health program in (a) school health services, (b) healthful school environment, and (c) health teaching); (3) to evaluate the learner in the areas of (a) knowledge, (b) attitudes and (c) behavior; and (4) to evaluate the teacher in (a) child-teacher interaction, and (b) methods used in health teaching.

Evaluation of health needs and interests is valuable in determining the types of services needed most by the school population and the type of instructional program that would be relevant to the greatest number of people in the school community to make the school-based instructional program more meaningful.

Evaluation of the overall school health program is necessary to direct attention to strengths and weaknesses of the total health program and to compare it with other programs. Priority can be given to identified areas of weakness. Even though the procedure is tedious and time-consuming, the effort is usually substantiated by the types of improvements that can be initiated. Improvements rationally based on data collected by means of evaluation often are accepted by administrators and school board members since the need can be substantiated.

Evaluation of the learner includes an assessment of the instructional program provided, the materials used to supplement the learning experiences and knowledge, and attitudes, and behaviors of the children.

In discussing the purposes of evaluation we find a need to evaluate all facets of the health program. There is need to include the teacher. During these times of accountability the responsible teacher will want to include a self-evaluation to measure the effectiveness of his or her input and guidance. As a facilitator of learning rather than an indoctrinator, the teacher will have data to help evaluate teaching methods, interactions with children and materials used to supplement health teaching.

There is much for children to learn in our modern society; therefore the time allowed for the school health program should be well spent. An evaluation well done and thoughtfully considered should result in better informed, more responsible children, more complete programs and more effective teachers.

EVALUATION OF THE SCHOOL HEALTH PROGRAM

The valuative measure applied will be determined by the phase of the total school health program being evaluated. Surveys, questionnaires, observations, class discussions and written tests can be used to assess whether or not, or how much the school health program is meeting the needs and interests of the children or particular community.

The evaluation of the *school health services* includes determining the thoroughness and frequency of physical examinations, vision and hearing screening, dental examinations and teacher observations of the children's health. The degree of success with follow-up programs should be assessed as well as the methods of prevention and control of communicable diseases, the extent of first aid provided within the school, and the management of emergency health treatment. In addition to qualified school administrators and staff, qualified community health department officials may be called to assist in the assessment of the school health services and certain aspects of the school environment.

The evaluation of the *school health environment* is perhaps the least difficult assessment of the total school health program. Sanitary facilities, for example, are static, and can be rated as adequate or inadequate or any place on a scale without a long-term evaluative process. Safety factors of the total school building and grounds are included as well as lighting, heating; ventilation; acoustics; fire-fighting equipment; size and type of desks and seating arrangements; noise level; frequency of interruptions; provision of healthful school climate afforded by teacher-child, child-child, teacher-teacher, and teacher-administration relationships. While the safety and adequacy of the school building is not difficult to assess, the healthful school climate that includes maintaining a psychological atmosphere that is most conducive to learning may be more difficult to evaluate.

In evaluating the instructional program which involves an assessment of child progress in health knowledge, attitudes and behavior, it is important to determine (1) what is being taught-relevancy of the curriculum, (2) when it is taught-realistic timing element according to the maturity level of children, and (3) how it is taught-effectiveness of teaching methods.

The following criteria can be applied to health teaching for purposes of evaluation.

1. Does the content meet the needs and interests of children?

2. Is the information accurate, honest and current?

3. Are the teaching methods effective and appropriate for the content and the ability of children?

4. Does the teaching method allow for the content learned through activities to be integrated into related experiences?

5. Does the teaching method allow for child investigation, interaction and internalization?

6. Are the objectives consistent with the concepts and subconcepts and basic understandings?

7. Are the objectives clearly stated in terms of behavioral expectations of the learner?

8. Are children given opportunity and encouraged to develop personal values that relate to health matters?

Evaluating knowledge is relatively simply compared to the evaluation of attitudes and behaviors. Within a given school system undoubtedly a variety of points of view will be held that influence children's attitudes. These may stem from cultural, ethnic or economical advantages or limitations. Attitudes can be evaluated by determining the value given a concept on a scale of one through five or one through seven. While this is not definitive, it is indicative of the children's attitudes about health.

EVALUATION OF THE LEARNER

To effectively evaluate the child it is important to develop baseline data. Only by knowing where children are at the beginning of a program is it possible to document and interpret the extent and direction of change in knowledge, attitudes and behaviors. These data can be obtained by pretesting and posttesting. With this information the teacher can adjust the program to include more emphasis in those areas where children show the greatest weakness. In areas where children show the greatest gaps of the content, the teacher may wish to guide them into more depth in the health area rather than omit it from the total health program. It is unlikely that the test scores of all children would show strongly the same weaknesses or strengths. But the scores can be valuable indicators of group needs, and important for identifying individual needs. The value of pretesting for individualized instruction is apparent. The periodic testing and evaluation of the child can be accomplished by the following.

1. Teacher-made written or oral objectives tests such as (a) multiple choice, (b) completion, (c) true and false or (d) matching.
2. Teacher-made written or oral subjective tests, such as (a) essays or discussion, (b) open ended stories, or (c) problem-solving situations.
3. Standardized tests (usually objective).
4. Interviews (subjective).
5. Questionnaire (subjective).
6. Self-appraisal (subjective).

TEACHER-MADE TESTS

Since one of the purposes of evaluation is to measure growth of the individual child in the areas of health, the teacher-made test is more likely to cover the information included in a particular topic than a standardized test. When teachers teach they want to see some evidence of growth. This growth can be seen to a certain extent in written evaluations.

However, written tests alone cannot adequately measure the three interrelated dimensions of health knowledge, health attitudes and health behavior. The child may be able to retain a considerable amount of knowledge concerning health, and the value of this knowledge cannot be underestimated in terms of lifelong effect on attitudes and practices. However, most teachers want to see evidence of growth in attitudes and behavior as well. Difficulties are often encountered in this type of evaluation. The evidence of growth in attitudes and behavior may not be demonstrated until the child is in a position to make more of his or her own decisions. For example, the child may have a good understanding of nutritional needs but until able to purchase and prepare his or her own food, attitudes may appear unchanged since there has been no observable change in behavior.

To obtain adequate measures of growth the teacher should include techniques to measure attitudes and behaviors as well as knowledge. Knowledge can be ascertained by (1) multiple-choice questions, (2) completion questions, (3) true and false questions or (4) matching questions. Attitudes and behaviors can be assessed by (1) written or oral essays of discussion, (2) open-ended stories or (3) decision-making situations. These subjective type tests require valid judgments on the part of the teacher.

Good test construction requires that the test items relate to the stated objectives. Each objective of a particular topical area should be considered and test items developed to evaluate the effectiveness of the activity and instruction provided to meet that specific objective. A teacher can then determine from the child responses the degree of effectiveness in motivating the learner. These test items, in addition to simple recall and recognition, should include other cognitive skills such as comprehension, analysis, appreciation, synthesis, internalization and decision-making. Therefore, for more complete assessment, the test design should be both objective and subjective since health content deals with the affective and action domains as well as the cognitive domain.

Test constructions also consider the objectivity, validity, reliability and practicality of the test items to make up the appraisal instrument. The test is objective if the child's score results are the same, regardless of the person who marked the test. The test is valid if it measures what it intends to measure. The test is reliable if essentially the same results are achieved when the test is repeated under the same conditions with similar groups. The test is considered practical if it produces the desired data, is appropriate for the ability level of the child, can be administered within the time range, and if the items are clearly stated. Test questions that confuse the child fail to provide an accurate measurement of the child's growth.

TEACHER COMPETENCIES

Teaching about health in today's society requires more than just an accurate knowledge of curriculum content. The competent, effective teacher recognizes that each child is a unique individual with capabilities and limitations. Individual differences make each child special. These differences challenge the teacher to create an atmosphere where interests are stimulated and children are helped to gain knowledge that will build wholesome attitudes and behaviors that will lead them to become all they are capable of becoming.

In order for teachers to be competent evaluators they must be competent teachers who feel good about themselves as persons, have confidence in their ability to guide children, possess an understanding of growth and development, have insight into the needs and interests of children, and have a mastery of the subject matter. The teacher must continue to develop as a person and continue to grow professionally. Teachers must continually review new methods of evaluation so that they can utilize the very best tools to measure child needs and growth and their own effectiveness.

TEACHER EVALUATIONS

The value of teacher evaluations cannot be minimized. Teachers should welcome this opportunity to further their understanding of themselves as persons and to grow professionally.

Teacher evaluations can be accomplished by (1) child-teacher evaluations, 92) teacher-behavior assessments, (3) videotaping and (4) audiotaping.

Teacher-behavior assessments may be completed at intervals by supervisors or peers. These assessments consider the teacher's behavior; interaction with children, peers and administrators; and methods of instruction. If the spirit of this type of evaluation is nonthreatening it can be a very effective tool for changing methods or behaviors which the teacher will recognize as harmful to children. If the behavior or method of instruction is not actually harmful, it may not be as effective as the teacher had perceived it to be. As a result of this evaluation, positive changes could be made that prove extremely important for both teacher and learner.

Videotape recordings have proved valuable in providing the teacher with an accurate feedback of teacher-child interaction and an opportunity for the teacher to observe his or her own teaching method. Videotapes can be observed along with a fellow teacher or supervisor who may be able to provide constructive suggestions.

Audiotape recordings can be helpful but lack the dimension of the videotape. Often, however, simply hearing a response and possibly identifying a pattern will provide insight and the stimulus to change an ineffective approach. From listening to recorded child responses, the teacher can often determine whether or not the objective is being met.

Child-teacher evaluations can be completed by the child, but are rarely used at the elementary school level. However, they can be simplified for child use and have value, especially at the 4-6 level.

None of these methods of teacher evaluation is complete in itself but can be used as an indicator in evaluating the instruction and the impact of the total program.

In this day of accountability, both within the school system and within the community, it is imperative that we use a sound evaluative program to improve curriculum design and teaching methods, and to answer questions raised by the community in regard to the school health program and its achievement.

All of the various evaluative procedures that have been suggested in this chapter have been used with varying degrees of success. It is hoped that they will provide useful guidelines for the reader, and that they will serve the purpose of helping individual teachers improve upon their own evaluative techniques.

SUGGESTIONS FOR SUPPLEMENTARY READING

Alvik, T., School-based evaluation: a close-up, *Studies in Educational Evaluation*, 21, March 1995, p. 311-43.

Barclay, K., and Benelli, C., Program evaluation through the eyes of a child, *Childhood Education*, 72, Winter 1995-96, p. 91-6.

Curran, R.R., Coercion and the ethics of grading and testing, *Educational Theory*, 45, Fall 1995, p. 425-41.

Garaway, G.B., Participatory evaluation, *Studies in Educational Evaluation*, 21, January 1995, p. 85-102.

Gathercoal, P. Principles of assessment, *Clearing House*, 69, September/October 1995, p. 59-61.

Israel, B.A., et al., Evaluation of health education programs; current assessment and future directions, *Health Education Quarterly*, 22, August 1995, p. 364-89.

McLellan, H., Evaluation in a situational learning environment, *Educational Technology Research and Development*, 34, March 1993, p. 39-45.

Nitko, A.J., Is the curriculum a reasonable basis for assessment reform? *Educational Measurement*, 14, Fall 1995, p. 5-10.

Van Reusen, K., and Robinson, J., Standards-based assessment in school health education, *Education*, 116, Summer 1996, p. 528-33.

Weston, C.B., A model for understanding formative evaluation in instructional design, *Educational Technology Research and Development*, 43, March 1995, p. 29-48.

TRAITS AND CHARACTERISTICS OF ELEMENTARY SCHOOL CHILDREN

FIVE-YEAR-OLD CHILDREN

PHYSICAL

1. Boys' height, 42 to 46 inches; weight, 38 to 49 pounds; girls' height, 42 to 46 inches; weight 36 to 48 pounds.
2. May grow two or three inches and gain from three to six pounds during the year.
3. Girls may be about a year ahead of boys in physiological development.
4. Beginning to have better control of body.
5. The large muscles are better developed than the small muscles that control the fingers and hands.
6. Usually determined whether he or she will be left-handed.
7. Eye and hand coordination is not complete.
8. May have farsighted vision.
9. Vigorous and noisy, but activity appears to have definite direction.
10. Tires easily and needs plenty of rest.
11. Can wash and take care of toilet needs.
12. Can use fork and spoon and may try to use knife.

SOCIAL

1. Interests in neighborhood games which involve any number of children.

2. Plays various games to test skill.
3. Enjoys other children and likes to be with them.
4. Interests are largely self-centered.
5. Seems to get along best in small groups.
6. Shows an interest in home activities.
7. Imitates when playing.
8. Gets along well in taking turns.
9. Respects the belongings of other people.

EMOTIONAL

1. Seldom shows jealousy toward younger siblings.
2. Usually sees only one way to do a thing.
3. Usually sees only one answer to a question.
4. Inclined not to change plans in the middle of an activity, but would rather begin over.
5. May fear being deprived of mother.
6. Some definite personality traits evidenced.
7. Is learning to get along better, but still may resort to quarreling and fighting.
8. Likes to be trusted with errands.
9. Enjoys performing simple tasks.
10. Wants to please and do what is expected.
11. Is beginning to sense right and wrong in terms of specific situations.

INTELLECTUAL

1. Enjoys copying designs, letters and numbers.
2. Interested in completing tasks.
3. May tend to monopolize table conversation.
4. Frequently bothered by frightening dreams.
5. Memory for past events good.
6. Looks at books and pretends to read them.
7. Likes recordings, words and music that tell a story.

8. Enjoys counting objects.
9. Over 2,000 words in vocabulary.
10. Can speak in complete sentences.
11. Can sing simple melodies, beat good rhythms and recognize simple tunes.
12. Daydreams seem to center around make-believe play.
13. Attention span increasing up to 20 minutes in some cases.
14. Is able to plan activities.
15. Enjoys stories, dramatic play and poems.
16. Enjoys making up dances to music.
17. Pronunciation is usually clear.
18. Can express needs well in words.

SIX-YEAR-OLD CHILDREN

PHYSICAL

1. Boys' height, 44 to 48 inches; weight, 41 to 54 pounds; girls' height, 43 to 48 inches, weight, 40 to 53 pounds.
2. Growth is gradual in weight and height.
3. Milk teeth shedding and first permanent molars emerging.
4. Good appetite and wants to eat between meals.
5. Good supply of energy.
6. Marked activity urge absorbed in running, jumping, chasing and dodging games.
7. Muscular control becoming more effective with large objects.
8. There is a noticeable change in the eye-hand behavior.
9. Legs lengthening rapidly.
10. Big muscles crave activity.

SOCIAL

1. Self-centered and has need for praise.
2. Likes to be first.
3. Indifferent to sex distinction.

4. Enjoys group play when groups tend to be small.
5. Likes parties but behavior may not always be decorous.
6. The majority enjoy school association and have a desire to learn.
7. Interested in conduct of friends.
8. Boys like to fight and wrestle with peers to prove masculinity.
9. Shows an interest in group approval.

EMOTIONAL

1. Restless and may have difficulty in making decisions.
2. Emotional pattern of anger may be difficult to control at times.
3. Behavior patterns may often be explosive and unpredictable.
4. Jealousy toward siblings at times; at other times takes pride in siblings.
5. Greatly excited by anything new.
6. Behavior becomes susceptible to shifts in direction, inwardly motivated and outwardly stimulated.
7. May be self-assertive and dramatic.

INTELLECTUAL

1. Vocabulary of over 2,500 words.
2. Interest span inclined to be short.
3. Knows number combinations making up to ten.
4. Knows comparative values of the common cons.
5. Can define simple objects in terms of what they are used for.
6. Knows right and left side of body.
7. Has an association with creative activity and motorized life experience.
8. Drawings are crude but realistic and suggestive of early man.
9. Will contribute to guided group planning.
10. Conversation usually concerns own experience and interests.
11. Curiosity is active and memory is strong.
12. Identifies with imaginary characters.

SEVEN-YEAR-OLD CHILDREN

PHYSICAL

1. Boys' height, 46 to 51 inches; weight, 45 to 60 pounds; girls' height 46 to 50 inches; weight, 44 to 59 pounds.
2. Big-muscle activity predominates in interest and value.
3. More improvement in eye-hand coordination.
4. May grow two or three inches and gain three to five pounds in weight during the year.
5. Tires easily and shows fatigue in the afternoon.
6. Has slow reaction time.
7. Needs to sleep approximately eleven hours daily on the average.
8. May have to be reminded at times about control of elimination.
9. Heart and lungs are smallest in proportion to body size.
10. General health may be precarious, with susceptibility to disease high and resistance low.
11. Endurance is relatively poor.
12. Coordination is improving with throwing and catching becoming more accurate.
13. Whole-body movements are under better control.
14. Small accessory muscles developing.
15. Displays amazing amounts of vitality.

SOCIAL

1. Wants recognition for individual achievements.
2. Sex differences are not of very great significance.
3. Not always a good loser.
4. Conversation often centers around family.
5. Learning to stand up for own rights.
6. Interested in friends and is not influenced by their social or economic status.
7. Attaining orientation in time.
8. Gets greater enjoyment from group play.

9. Shows greater signs of cooperative efforts.

EMOTIONAL

1. Curiosity and creative desires may condition responses.
2. May be difficult to take criticism from adults.
3. Wants to be more independent.
4. Reaching for new experiences and trying to relate to enlarged world.
5. Over anxious to reach goals set by parents and teachers.
6. Critical of self and sensitive to failure.
7. Emotional pattern of anger is more controlled.
8. Becoming less impulsive and boisterous in actions that at six.

INTELLECTUAL

1. Abstract thinking is barely beginning.
2. Is able to listen longer.
3. Is able to reason, but has little experience upon which to base judgments.
4. The attention span is still short and retention poor, but does not object to repetition.
5. Reaction time is still slow.
6. Learning to evaluate the achievements of self and others.
7. Concerned with own lack of skill and achievement.
8. Becoming more realistic and less imaginative.

EIGHT-YEAR-OLD CHILDREN

PHYSICAL

1. Boys' height, 48 to 53 inches; weight, 49 to 70 pounds; girls' height, 48 to 52 inches; weight, 47 to 66 pounds.
2. Interested in activities requiring coordination of small muscles.
3. Arms are lengthening and hands are growing larger.

4. Eyes can accommodate more easily.
5. Some develop poor posture.
6. Accidents appear to occur more frequently at this age.
7. Fewer communicable diseases.
8. Appreciates correct skill performance.

SOCIAL

1. Girls are more careful about their clothes than boys.
2. Leaves many things uncompleted.
3. Has special friends.
4. Has longer periods of peaceful play.
5. Does not like playing alone.
6. Enjoys dramatizing.
7. Starts collections.
8. Enjoys school and dislikes staying home.
9. Likes variety.
10. Recognition of property rights is well established.
11. Responds well to group activity.
12. Interest will focus on friends of own sex.
13. Beginning of the desire to become a member of the club.

EMOTIONAL

1. Dislikes taking much criticism from adults.
2. Can give and take criticism in own group.
3. May develop enemies.
4. Does not like to be treated as a child.
5. Has a marked sense of humor.
6. First impulse is to blame others.

INTELLECTUAL

1. Can tell day of month and year.
2. Voluntary attention span increasing.
3. Interested in far-off places, and ways of communication now have real meaning.
4. Becoming more aware of adult world and place in it.
5. Ready to tackle almost anything.
6. Shows a capacity for self-evaluation.
7. Likes to memorize.
8. Not always too good at telling time, but very much aware of it.

NINE-YEAR-OLD CHILDREN

PHYSICAL

1. Boys' height, 50 to 55 inches; weight, 55 to 74 pounds, girls' height, 50 to 54 inches; weight 52 to 74 pounds.
2. Increasing strength in arms, hands and fingers.
3. Endurance improving.
4. Needs and enjoys much activity; boys like to shout, wrestle and tussle with each other.
5. A few girls near puberty.
6. Girls' growth maturity gaining over boys' up to two years.
7. Girls enjoy being active, but are usually less noisy and less full of spontaneous energy than boys.
8. Likely to slouch and assume unusual posture.
9. Eyes are much better developed and are able to accommodate with less strain.
10. Needs ten to eleven hours sleep on the average; is a good sleeper, but often does not get enough sleep.
11. Sex differences appear in recreational activities.
12. Interested in own body and wants to have questions answered.

SOCIAL

1. Wants to be like others, talk like others and look like them.
2. Girls are becoming more interested in their clothes.
3. Is generally a conformist and may be afraid of that which is different.
4. Less dependent on others.
5. Able to be fairly responsible and dependable.
6. Some firm and loyal friendships may develop.
7. Increasing development of qualities of leadership and followership.
8. Increasing interest in activities involving challenges and adventure.
9. Increasing participation in varied and organized group activities.

EMOTIONAL

1. May sometimes be outspoken and critical of adults, although there is a genuine fondness for them.
2. Responds best to adults when treated as an individual and approached in an adult way.
3. Likes recognition for what has been done and responds well to deserved praise.
4. Likely to be backward about public recognition, but likes private praise.
5. Developing sympathy and loyalty to others.
6. Does not mind criticism or punishment if it is fair, but is indignant if it is unfair.
7. Disdainful of danger to and safety, which may be a result of increasing interest in activities involving challenges and adventure.

INTELLECTUAL

1. Individual differences are clear and distinct.
2. Some real interests are beginning to develop.
3. Beginning to have a strong sense of right and wrong.
4. Understands explanations.

5. Interests are closer to ten or eleven-year-olds than to seven or eight-year-olds.
6. As soon as a project fails to hold interest, it may be dropped without further thought.
7. Attention span is greatly increased.
8. Seems to be guided best by a reason, simple and clear-cut, for a decision which needs to be made.
9. Ready to learn from occasional failure of judgment as long as learning takes place in situations where failure will not have too serious consequences.
10. Able to make up own mind and come to decisions.
11. Marked reading disabilities begin to be more evident and may tend to influence the personality.
12. Range of interest in reading in that many are great readers while others may be barely interested in books.
13. Will average between six and seven words per remark.

TEN-YEAR-OLD CHILDREN

PHYSICAL

1. Boys' height, 52 to 57 inches; weight, 59 to 82 pounds; girls' height, 52 to 57 inches; weight 57 to 83 pounds.
2. Individuality is well defined and insights are more mature.
3. Stability in growth rate and stability of physiological processes.
4. Physically active and likes to rush around and be busy.
5. Before the onset of puberty there is usually a resting period or plateau, during which boys or girls do not appear to gain in either height or weight.
6. Interested in the development of more skills.
7. Reaction time is improving.
8. Muscular strength does not seem to keep pace with growth.
9. Refining and elaborating skill in the use of small muscles.

SOCIAL

1. Begins to recognize the fallibility of adults.
2. Moving more into a peer-centered society.
3. Both boys and girls are amazingly self-dependent.
4. Self-reliance has grown, and at the same time intensified group feelings are required.
5. Divergence between the two sexes is widening.
6. Great team loyalties are developing.
7. Beginning to identify with one's social contemporaries of the same sex.
8. On the whole has a fairly critical sense of justice.
9. Boys show their friendship with other boys by wrestling and jostling with each other, while girls walk around with arms around each other as friends.
10. Interest in people in the community and in affairs of some world events may be keen.
11. Interested in social problems in an elementary way and likes to take part in discussions.

EMOTIONAL

1. Increasing tendency to rebel against adult domination.
2. Capable of loyalties and hero worship, and can inspire it in schoolmates.
3. Can be readily inspired to group loyalties in club organization.
4. Likes the sense of solidarity which comes from keeping a group secret as a member of a group.
5. Each sex has an increasing tendency to show lack of sympathy and understanding with the other.
6. Boys' and girls' behavior and interests becoming increasingly different.

INTELLECTUAL

1. Works with executive speed and likes the challenge of mathematics.
2. Shows a capacity to budget time and energy.

3. Can attend to a visual task and at the same time maintain conversation.
4. Some become discouraged and may give up trying when unsuccessful.
5. The attention span has lengthened considerably, with the child able to listen to and follow directions and retain knowledge more easily.
6. Beginning understanding of real casual relations.
7. Making finer conceptual distinctions and thinking reflectively.
8. Developing scientific approach.
9. Better oriented with respect to time.
10. Ready to plan the day and accept responsibility for getting things done on time.

ELEVEN-YEAR-OLD CHILDREN

PHYSICAL

1. Boys' height, 53 to 58 inches; weight, 64 to 91 pounds; girls' height, 53 to 59 inches; weight, 64 to 95 pounds.
2. Marked changes in muscular system causing awkwardness and habits sometimes distressing to the child.
3. Shows fatigue more easily.
4. Some girls and a few boys suddenly show rapid growth and evidence of the approach of adolescence.
5. In general this is a period of good health with fewer diseases and infections.
6. On the average girls may be taller and heavier than boys.
7. Uneven growth of different parts of the body.
8. Rapid growth may result in laziness in the lateral type of child, and fatigue and irritability of the linear type.
9. Willing to work hard at acquiring physical skills, and emphasis is on excellence of performance of physical feats.
10. Boys are more active and rough in games than girls.
11. Eye-hand coordination well developed.
12. Bodily growth is more rapid than heart growth, and lungs are not fully developed.
13. Boys develop greater power in shoulder girdle and lungs.

SOCIAL

1. Internal guiding standards have been set up and, although guided by what is done by other children, will modify behavior in line with those standards already set up.
2. Does a number of socially acceptable things not because they are right or wrong.
3. Although obsessed by standards of peers, is anxious for social approval from adults.
4. Need for social life companionship of children of own age.
5. Liking for organized games more and more prominent.
6. Girls are likely to be self-conscious in the presence of boys and are usually much more mature than boys.
7. Team spirit is very strong.
8. Boys' and girls' interests are not always the same and there may be some antagonism between the sexes.
9. Often engages in silly behavior, such as giggling and clowning.
10. Girls are more interested in social appearance than are boys.

EMOTIONAL

1. If unskilled in group games and game skills, may tend to withdraw.
2. Boys may be concerned if they feel they are underdeveloped.
3. May appear to be indifferent and uncooperative.
4. Moods change quickly.
5. Wants to grow up, but may be afraid to leave childhood security behind.
6. Increase in self-direction and in a serious attitude toward work.
7. Need for approval to feel secure.
8. Beginning to have a fully developed idea of own importance.

INTELLECTUAL

1. Increasing power of attention and abstract reasoning.

2. Able to maintain a longer period of intellectual activity between firsthand experiences.
3. Interested in scientific experiences and procedures.
4. Can carry on many individual intellectual responsibilities.
5. Able to discuss problems and to see different sides of questions.
6. May lack maturity of judgment.
7. Increased language facility.
8. Attention span is increasing and concentration may be given to a task for a long period of time.
9. Level of aspiration has increased.
10. Growing in ability to use several facts to make a decision.
11. Insight into casual relationships is developing more and is manifested by many why and how questions.

TWELVE-YEAR-OLD CHILDREN

PHYSICAL

1. Boys' height, 55 to 61 inches; weight, 70 to 101 pounds; girls' height, 56 to 62 inches; weight, 72 to 107 pounds.
2. Becoming more skillful in the use of small muscles.
3. May be relatively little body change in some cases.
4. Ten hours of sleep is considered average.
5. Heart rate at rest is between 80 and 90.

SOCIAL

1. Increasing identification of self with other children of own sex.
2. Increasing recognition of fallibility of adults.
3. May see self as a child and adults as adults.
4. Getting ready to make the difficult transition to adolescence.
5. Pressure is being placed on individual at this level to begin to assume adult responsibilities.

EMOTIONAL

1. Beginning to develop a truer picture of morality.
2. Clearer understanding of real causal relations.
3. The process of sexual maturation involves structural and physiological changes with possible perplexing and disturbing emotional problems.
4. Personal appearance may become a source of great conflict, and learning to appreciate good grooming or the reverse may be prevalent.
5. May be very easily hurt when criticized or made the scapegoat.
6. Mal-adjustments may occur when there is not a harmonious relationship between child and adult.

INTELLECTUAL

1. Learns more ways of studying and controlling the physical world.
2. The use of language (on many occasions his or her own vocabulary) to exchange ides or for explanatory reasons.
3. More use of reflective thinking and greater ease of distinction.
4. Continuation in development of scientific approach.

INDEX

S

safety education, 50, 58
school curriculum, 5, 7, 35, 47, 195
school health program, 5, 17, 18, 19, 24, 25, 46, 211, 212, 213, 214, 219
School health service, 18
screening tests, 37
Self-Testing Activities, 179
Seven-Year-Old Children, 225
sex education, 50, 61, 87, 89, 90, 96, 97, 98, 99
Six-Year-Old Children, 223
social studies, 5, 39, 78, 116, 145, 159, 160, 161, 162, 169, 172, 173, 195
Speech defects, 23
submarines, 153

T

Teachers, Qualifications of, 26
Teaching methods, 67
team games, 28, 176, 177, 185

television commercials, 53, 57, 78
Ten-Year-Old Children, 230
Theory of Active Game Learning, 180
three-dimensional construction, 199
Twelve-Year-Old Children, 234

U

Unit Teaching, 161
United States, 5, 169, 199

V

verbal learning, 180, 184
Vermont, 199
visual defects, 21

W

Whitney, Eli, 171
word-recognition, 114, 115